From Autism to Alzheimer's and Everything in Between

How to Fix the Brain Using the Restoration Model

From Autism to Alzheimer's and Everything in Between

How to Fix the Brain Using the Restoration Model

By Jean-Ronel Corbier, MD

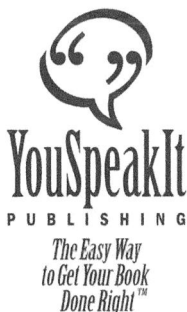

YouSpeakIt
PUBLISHING
*The Easy Way
to Get Your Book
Done Right*™

www.YouSpeakItPublishing.com

ISBN: 978-1-945446-24-5

Dedication

Dedicated to all my past, present, and future patients, to anyone looking for brain restoration and healing, and to my family and friends for all of their love and support.

Acknowledgments

Writing a book is like building a house. It takes a good plan, a great deal of preparation, and the work of people with a variety of skills. During the writing of this book, I have received support and have drawn inspiration from many.

I would like to offer my heartfelt thanks to the following people:

To my staff at the Brain Restoration Clinic, a division of the Integra Wellness Center: Rebekah, Rebecca, Jocelyn, Lesa, and Hannah, for putting up with me while writing the book, despite being very busy at the office.

To the many parents who have inspired me with their persistence and tenacity on behalf of their children, including:

Joyce and Brian Wulf, who were told that their newborn son, Matthew, had six to twelve months to live, but decided to fight even though this meant travelling overseas at least eighteen times to get answers. Matthew, now eighteen, is himself the recent author of a book.

Fred and Karen Callahan, parents of an autistic child, Cal, who are determined to support research until a cure for autism is found, whatever it takes. They are persistent and patient problem solvers.

Melanie and Rob Gentile, parents of Maria, a child with Rett syndrome, who are devoted parents and steadfast fighters. They have never given up, even when times were very rough.

It has been my privilege to partner with parents like these. Undeterred by the setbacks they have weathered in the past, they have inspired me with their devotion to finding effective, innovative, safe, and affordable solutions for their children. Parents like the ones mentioned above can form uniquely effective research teams as well.

Finally, thank you to Keith Leon, as well as Cameron, Nida, and the rest of the staff at YouSpeakIt Publishing for helping a busy physician like me get this work into physical form in a seamless and enjoyable manner.

Contents

Introduction

As a neurologist, I have spent years studying the brain and the rest of the nervous system. I have encountered many hard-to-treat neurological disorders and, over time, I have discovered that these disorders can be treated successfully using the right approach.

This book highlights a variety of common but complex disorders that affect children as well as adults. You will read about a specialized approach to patient care that I have developed and how it can be applied to bring patients back to health.

If you or a loved one are suffering from a chronic disorder, and you are feeling frustrated, I urge you not to give up!

My goal in writing this book is to reach out to the many people who are sick and suffering, to explain how they can beat their illness even if they have already seen specialists and have been told that nothing else could be done.

Often in my practice, I see patients who, along with their parents and family, have been dealing with a medical problem for a long time. Sometimes, if the problem is very complex, they may have already seen a variety of specialists or have gone to elite medical centers where tertiary care is provided, yet they continue to suffer with their problems.

When I evaluate these patients, I often see that the approach that has been used to treat them has not been comprehensive or integrative enough. Instead of getting to the core of the problem, sometimes their treatment plan has been solely focused on addressing symptoms.

I decided to write this book to introduce a specific approach — one that is very broad and methodical — that can get to the root cause of the problems. In my experience, this is how true healing — which I define as the restoration of healthy functioning — can occur. I call this approach the Restoration Model.

In this book, I will discuss brain and neurological conditions like autism, a condition I have treated in many hundreds of children over the past decade and a half, and PANDAS (Pediatric Autoimmune Neuropsychiatric Disorders Associated with Streptococcal Infections), which is another childhood disorder involving the brain and the immune system. I will also discuss several adult-onset disorders, including Alzheimer's disease.

While highlighting different disorders in each chapter, we will explore together such concepts as the *three brains*, the gut-brain connection, and the mind-body interactions that influence various aspects of health and healing. You will learn about functional illnesses like fibromyalgia, and neuroimmune conditions masquerading — and misdiagnosed — as psychiatric illness.

There are five chapters in this book, and each chapter will focus on a particular type of condition. These conditions have been chosen because they allow me to present an important set of concepts that make specific points about health and healing.

I have chosen disorders that are common. You or your loved one may, in fact, be suffering from one of these disruptive disorders. If that is the case, I would like you to understand that help is available, and that suffering does not have to continue.

The suggestions made in each chapter can be applied to other complex conditions as well, even if they are not specifically mentioned in the book.

Each of the medical conditions discussed is representative of a class of disorders. You will find that the discussions emphasize particular concepts — such as detoxification, inflammation, and antioxidant function — that apply to that kind of disorder. However, most of these concepts can be readily applied to other disorders as well. You will find that certain concepts and principles are repeated several times throughout the book, which reflect their importance.

If you are particularly interested in a disorder mentioned in one of the chapters, it is perfectly okay to start with that chapter out of interest, but be sure to read the other chapters as well.

I recommend reading each chapter carefully, even if it highlights an issue that you may be less interested in. You may pick up some unexpected pearls of wisdom that apply directly to your own health issues. The discussions in each chapter will also emphasize some important concepts that pertain to brain healing in general.

This book is not meant to replace the care you are given by your own health providers, but will hopefully enhance your medical experience, and perhaps stimulate you to ask appropriate questions at your clinical appointments. When it comes to your health, it is always good to learn everything you can.

If you are suffering with a condition for which treatment has been unsuccessful, this book will offer you some alternatives to consider. Approaching your problem from a more holistic and integrative angle may be the key to successful treatment and a restoration of your health in body and mind.

The main message I would like you to get from this book is that no matter how chronic and complex a medical condition may appear, there is still hope. Don't give up!

Healing is always possible.

CHAPTER ONE

Autism
The Disorder of the Century

AUTISM IS A COMPLEX AND ENIGMATIC NEU-ROLOGICAL DISORDER

I am a board-certified neurologist with special qualifications in child neurology. I work with both children and adult patients. Of all the neurological conditions that I work with, I have found that autism — by far — is the most intriguing and complex.

Children with autism suffer simultaneously from a large variety of disturbances that disrupt the fabric of the mind, the brain, and the body in a remarkable way. Simply put, when it comes to autism, think of *dysregulation:* a breakdown in the regulation of normal processes.

Autistic children may exhibit forms of dysregulation in many areas, including:

- Mood
- Emotions

- Behavior
- Social interaction
- Language
- Bowel function
- Sensory input
- Movement
- Immune function

Dysregulation in just one of these areas can cause problems that can greatly affect quality of life. Imagine a child who becomes miserable when hearing a particular sound. You may not even notice the sound, but for this child, it is overwhelming. Now imagine the child simultaneously experiencing the results of dysregulation in several of the other areas listed above, and then you can begin to appreciate why an autistic child's behavior may be erratic. It is easy to understand why meltdowns may occur frequently.

The set of symptoms of autism in a child will not only affect the child, but also the child's family, classmates, and other people in the child's life. Because of this, developing a full understanding of autism requires transcending the fields of biology and medicine. One must also consider psychosocial factors, economics, and even deeper philosophical and spiritual questions.

Autism Is a Multifactorial Condition

What is autism?

Autism is a neurodevelopmental disorder in children. It is usually diagnosed before the age of three and is generally characterized by abnormalities in three main areas:

1. There is impairment in language and communication.

2. There are dysfunctions pertaining to behavior.

3. There are problems with social interaction.

In addition, sensory disturbances are typically present. To complicate matters, an important subset of children with autism appear normal at the onset but then regress and go on to develop symptoms.

Autism disorders exist on a spectrum that ranges from mild to severe, hence the term *autistic spectrum disorder*, often abbreviated ASD.

Listed below are some characteristics of children with autism on the severe end of the spectrum:

- Children may be nonverbal, non-communicative, or non-interactive socially.

- Some may be very sensitive to sounds.

- Some children may not be able to tolerate touch at all; contact may provoke tantrum behavior.

- There may be unusual repetitive movements such as hand flapping, jumping, and toe walking.

- Some children may make repetitive sounds like "eee".

- Children with autism may seem self-absorbed and cut off from their external environment.

- Sometimes, significant cognitive impairments go along with the autistic symptoms.

- Regarding health, the child may struggle with constipation or diarrhea, or may have chronic health issues such as multiple ear infections.

- Some are very picky eaters or may select foods in a strange fashion; for instance, they may avoid foods of a certain color or shape or be intolerant of certain mixtures.

On the other end of the spectrum, a child with autism can have a very high IQ, and some may only have minor behavioral issues. Some may be verbal with a strong vocabulary — though there may be oddities when it comes to inflection of voice or scope of conversations.

The Search for the Causes of Autism

Much of my professional career has been devoted to the task of trying to decipher and unravel the mysteries — and there are many — surrounding the multifaceted, chronic disorder that we call autism, the disorder of the century.

What causes autism?

The question is a difficult one to answer. What is interesting about autism is the fact that there is no one single cause for this complex disorder. Instead, there are many different possible etiologies. You might in fact refer to *autisms* instead of *autism* since there are so many different underlying causes.

Proposed causative factors include:

- Neurometabolic disorders
- Viral infections
- Genetic factors
- Environmental toxins

Neurometabolic disorders are conditions or dysfunctions in the metabolic processing system of the body. Two examples are phenylketonuria (PKU) and mitochondrial disorder. These kinds of disorders (i.e. neurometabolic conditions as a whole) are found in an important subset of children with autism. In addition, certain types of viral infections, like Rubella and herpes simplex virus (HSV), have been linked to the development of autism.

Genetics may be a factor that can predispose a person to the development of autism. There is no single *autism gene*, but a variety of different genes that could trigger the development of autism.

Often, genetic mutations may work hand in hand with environmental triggers, like toxins, that interact with the gene in such a way as to disrupt the circuitry of the brain, leading to autism. If a child also has the inability to properly rid the body of the toxin via a detoxification mechanism, this can spell more trouble.

In addition to a gene-environment interaction, we must also factor in timing; the interactions must occur at just the right time to have an effect. Autism symptoms usually appear early, during a time when the developing brain is very vulnerable to outside attacks.

There are, therefore, a variety of factors that must come together at the right time and in the right order to cause the changes that lead to autism. Another way to state this is to say that there are sets of circumstances that follow a specific sequence that, in a predisposed child, can result in autism. This same kind of mechanism may apply to conditions like attention deficit hyperactive disorder (ADHD) and Tourette's syndrome.

There Is an Epidemic Rise in the Diagnosis of Autism

Why is the number of patients increasing?

I started working in the field of autism in 2000. At that time, I was already amazed that the incidence of autism in the United States was one out of every 166 children. And then, a couple years later, the incidence of autism rose to one out of every 150 children. When you look at these numbers, consider the fact that, just a few decades ago, autism was considered a rare disorder, and the incidence was only one in ten thousand.

Unfortunately, that trend has continued. In 2007, the Centers for Disease Control and Prevention (CDC) released the prevalence report that one in 150 children in the United States had autism. Then, according to the CDC, about one in sixty-eight or 1.5 percent of children were identified with ASD based on tracking in eleven communities across the United States in 2012. On March 31, 2016, the CDC released its latest autism prevalence report showing that the prevalence among the nation's children remained unchanged, at one in sixty-eight. Although unchanged, the latest report also showed that less than half of autistic children (only 43 percent) were evaluated for developmental concerns by the age of three. This is a problem, since autism can be diagnosed today as early as age two. For the full scientific report, see the following link: cdc.gov/mmwr/volumes/65/ss/ss6503a1.htm.

What is the cause of this dramatic rise in autism?

The following ideas have been proposed in recent years:

- Both parents and doctors have become more familiar with the symptoms of autism, and this increases the likelihood of diagnosis.

- Due to increased knowledge and publicity, *diagnostic substitutions* may be on the rise. These occur when the diagnosis of one disorder is made — in this case, autism — for symptoms that would have been labeled differently in previous years.

- Special labeling for the condition of autism may have increased the likelihood that parents seek a medical diagnosis so their children can qualify for assistance and educational benefits.

There is no doubt that these changes have played a role in the increased diagnosing of autism. However, these factors alone are not enough to explain the exponential rise in autism.

In the past, genetics was believed to be the main culprit. There are certainly genetic influences; however, genetics alone cannot explain the steep increase in autism. We must therefore look at environmental factors as contributors to the development of autism.

But the question is, how do we identify what all the various environmental triggers are?

And how do we deconstruct the gene-environment interaction as it pertains to the rise in autism?

To this day, there is still no clear answer to these all-important questions.

Clinicians and researchers in the field continue to look for the answers. We already have made some great strides, but there is much more work to be done.

There Are Specific Ailments Pertaining to Autism That Give Us Important Clues

When I first started working with autism, parents would come to me and say, "Dr. Corbier, you are a child neurologist, and we have a child on the autism spectrum. What can you do to help?"

They would usually preface this by telling me that they'd already seen several specialists.

Typically, the parents who came to me were especially concerned about their child's lack of ability to communicate with others. Often, the child's speech was very limited, or in some cases, nonexistent.

When I was new to the field, I did some research to see what could be done to help kids who were significantly afflicted with speech and language delays. I also looked for ways to treat other conditions, such as neurobehavioral problems, that were not responding to any of the common treatments — therapies, counseling, or medications.

Initially, I was surprised to see that there were no readily found answers to these kinds of problems. There were ways of managing the symptoms, but there was no real way of coming up with a cure for these patients.

It was clear that our aim should not be to mask symptoms, but to restore proper functioning for these children. To do this, we needed to get to the root causes of the problems.

I eventually developed a model to work by — the Restoration Model — that seeks to look at the underlying sets of problems that exist, so that we can come up with a deep solution to restore brain function, whether it pertains to restoration of speech and language, behavior, processing problems, or the variety of other conditions that may be refractory to common treatments.

When autism — or another neurodevelopmental condition — appears hard to treat, this tells us that we are not using the right approach. Often, the answers can be found by using a broader, more holistic approach. This is what the Restoration Model provides.

Over the years, I started to look at nutrition for the nervous system, and I found that, in some cases, simply correcting the diet would have a profound effect on various neurological functions, such as speech, behavior, and sensory processing. I started to find that gastrointestinal dysfunction, as well as immune dysfunction, had a direct impact on cognition and behavior. I also became convinced that environmental toxins played a big role, since removing them made a big difference in several cases.

I firmly believe that, with the right approach, we can always find a way to successfully treat a patient. Focusing on autism, I began to develop a unique approach to treatment that could be effective for such a complex disorder.

UNDERSTANDING AUTISM CAN YIELD VALU-ABLE LESSONS

As a child neurologist working with autism, I was determined to come up with specific solutions. I found that by taking the time to research and fully assess the underlying factors that are present, we could then develop precisely the right interventions for a patient. Then, working persistently, we could successfully address the problems.

My goal was to lead the patient with autism to an improved quality of life by improving behavior, cognitive function, language, and other areas of dysfunction.

Before I started working with children with autism, I wanted to learn everything I could about the brain. I spent many years in training in order to attempt to understand the various mechanisms of the brain. My search took me to multiple institutions, including the University of Cincinnati, the Children's Hospital of Cincinnati, Johns Hopkins Medical School, and the Mayo Clinic.

However, when I actually started working with kids with autism, I found that just understanding the brain—as important as that was—was not sufficient. I needed to look at other organ systems in the body.

The Three Brains

The term *brain* refers to the control center of your body. However, for patients with neurological disorders, it is useful to broaden your view so that it reflects the complexity of the body. Functionally, we have not just one, but *three* brains:

1. We have a brain inside our skull that I call the *intra-cranial brain*. This is the brain that I spent all those years studying in school.

2. We have a brain inside of our gut that I call the *intra-abdominal brain*. It consists of more than one hundred million nerve cells responsible for the control and regulation of our digestive system. There is a medical field known as neuroenterology that is entirely focused on the connection between the gut and the nervous system.

3. The third brain is the one I refer to as the *floating brain*. It is also known as the immune system.

The interaction between these three brains adds to the complexity of neurological issues. Exploring the interplay between these control systems is an integral part of the Restoration Model. It enables doctor and patient to gain a more complete understanding of the condition of the whole body so that an appropriate treatment can be devised.

These three control centers are vital for regulation of your body processes. If dysfunctional conditions exist in the control centers — as often occurs in cases of autism and other neurological disorders — they can have an enormous impact on the operation of the body. It is valuable to study how these three brains talk to each other and support each other, but also to understand how these forces can cause massive damage to the body when something goes wrong.

Autism and the Gut-Brain Connection

Many children with autism have gastrointestinal abnormalities that need evaluation.

Common gastrointestinal issues include:

- Pain
- Reflux
- Spitting up
- Diarrhea
- Constipation
- Bloating

These kids often suffer tremendously, and their gastrointestinal discomfort may play a significant role in setting off some of the mysterious behavioral difficulties these patients exhibit.

Over the years, researchers have discovered that children with autism have a variety of pathologies of the gut that cause not only pain and discomfort, but also cause changes in neurologic function and behavior. Note that the interaction between the *intra-cranial brain* and the *intra-abdominal brain* is clearly a factor in these cases.

Please see the following links showing research data pertaining to autism and the gut-brain connection:

ncbi.nlm.nih.gov/pmc/articles/PMC4698498 and poo
.caltech.edu/static/pdf/Gastrointestinal_Issues_in_
Autism_Spectrum.5.pdf.

Many children have a condition called *leaky gut
syndrome.* Normally, tight junctions in the lining of the
gut keep unwanted substances from leaking into the
bloodstream. In a patient with leaky gut syndrome,
the tight junctions have become compromised. It is
especially common in patients with gluten sensitivity.
Leaky gut syndrome is associated with all sorts of
problems; the ones that catch my attention are those
that impact the brain.

There are numerous illustrations of the gut-brain
connection; it can clearly be seen in the progression and
symptoms of many medical conditions. Gut disorders
can have neurological impact, and conversely, some
neurological disorders can have associated gut
symptoms.

Some examples are listed below:

- The same processes that can lead to leaky gut
  syndrome can also cause *leaky brain syndrome.*
  The blood-brain barrier is designed to protect
  the brain from outside influences but, like the
  tight junctions in the gut, this too can become
  impaired or leaky.

- It is known that individuals with gluten allergies, as in the case of celiac disease, may suffer not only from gut issues, but also neurological problems such as *gluten ataxia*, which results in an unsteady gait. They may have hard-to-control seizures and a whole host of other neurological impairments.

- Abnormalities in the gastrointestinal system like the *gluten enteropathy*, described above, can secondarily affect the brain and cause *gluten encephalopathy*, which causes symptoms like brain fog, confusion, and irritability.

- Abdominal pain, nausea, or vomiting commonly accompany migraine headaches.

- An abnormal gut sensation or *aura* often precedes an epileptic seizure.

- Anxiety often presents with psychosomatic gastrointestinal symptoms that may be described as a *nervous stomach*.

In fact, clinical studies show that there may be a connection between peptic ulcers and anxiety disorder. See the following link: ncbi.nlm.nih.gov/pubmed/23453387.

Understanding how gut issues can influence the brain is a key element to designing a treatment plan for patients with autism. When I am treating a child with autism, I find myself spending as much time addressing gastrointestinal issues as I do discussing neurological issues. Tackling the gut issues from the beginning can completely change the quality of life for a child with autism.

Autism and the Brain-Immune Connection

Remember the three brains we discussed early in this chapter?

The previous section was related to the second brain, the intra-abdominal brain. This section is about the third brain, the floating brain: the immune system. Understanding the brain-immune connection is vital to an understanding of autism and related conditions, as is the gut-brain connection.

The immune system has memory, is intelligent, and is intricately and intimately linked to the nervous system. In fact, the immune system interacts not just with the brain, but also with the *mind*, which is composed of our conscious and unconscious selves. What we think and how we feel can impact the nervous system, which in turn can affect the immune system. The field of psychoneuroimmunology is devoted to the study of these interactions.

Researchers have found that, in the brains of children with autism, there is localized immune dysfunction, as well as inflammation. If treatment can successfully address these problems, substantial improvement in patient symptoms may occur. In fact, one of the treatment modalities that has a dramatic effect on some children with autism involves an intervention that modulates the immune system.

The following link pertains to a John Hopkins study (in collaboration with the University of Alabama) representing the largest RNA sequencing of autism brains, showing a clear link between innate immunity and neuronal activity in the etiology of autism (nature. com/articles/ncomms6748).

Researchers have found that up to one-third of individuals with psychiatric conditions such as depression and mood disorders also have immunological disturbances (jamanetwork.com/ journals/jamapsychiatry/fullarticle/1696348). Many of these individuals who do not respond to conventional antidepressant medications may respond to immunological treatments.

Autism: Genetic and Environmental Factors

The gene-environment interaction is a strong factor in the development of autism. One may be predisposed to autism because of certain genes, but not necessarily destined to develop symptoms. The development of symptoms may be dependent on the presence or absence of certain environmental triggers. Because we have more control over our environment than our genes, we must seize the opportunity to remove harmful environmental triggers from the autism equation as much as possible.

Even genetic expression itself can be altered through lifestyle. Many genes that are present in an individual are unexpressed — dormant — until they are stimulated in some way. Researchers in this field — called *epigenetics* — study the mechanisms of turning genes on and off. If we can manipulate genetic expression as well as environmental triggers; then we have a shot at reversing autism symptoms. The earlier that one intervenes, the better. As mentioned elsewhere in the book, timing is key when it comes to the development of autism. Early intervention matters.

Based on the understanding above, in my practice, each patient's genetic profile is evaluated and potential environmental triggers are assessed.

I spend time evaluating every patient's genetic profile, because this can yield valuable information. After all, we're all unique, so personalized or individualized medicine is the most effective strategy. I also do my best to identify the various environmental or outside triggers that can affect a patient.

Your unique genetic profile can dictate how you process or interact with your environment. This means that environmental triggers can affect individuals in different ways.

Most people, for instance, have the ability to get rid of toxins that we are exposed to. However, if you have a genetic mutation or alteration, you may not be able to process certain toxins properly. Knowing this information in advance can allow us to fine-tune our treatment approach, so that we can help every individual process environmental triggers more effectively.

Gathering this information is an essential part of our Restoration Model. Analyzing each patient's genetic tendencies and potential triggers can play a big role in restoring proper function.

Although autism appears enigmatic, we know that there is a combination of both genetic and environmental factors that are at play. The more we can explain this link, the better off we will be when it comes to an understanding of autism and other related conditions.

AUTISM AND THE RESTORATION MODEL

Autism is perhaps the most complex disorder that I know of as a physician, because it involves so many different factors, not only pertaining to the biological abnormalities that are present, but also psychological, social, and even spiritual elements.

The latter may not often be discussed, but are very important; as humans, we are made up of mind, body, and *spirit*.

According to our Restoration Model, healing is possible, but only if one acknowledges and addresses simultaneously factors that fall in the biological, psychological, social, and spiritual realms. Autism lends itself very well to this model, as it is a multifaceted, multifactorial, and multidimensional condition.

There Are Various Brain Dysfunctions Present in Autism

To properly address autism and to treat the various dysfunctions that are present, we must start with a clear understanding of the clinical or biological aspects of autism.

Certain portions of the brain appear to be underdeveloped in autistic patients, while others are overdeveloped. There are connectivity abnormalities in the brain that affect not just one part of the brain; they affect neural networks that connect different parts of the brain.

As I have mentioned above, autism is a problem of dysregulation, and in the brain, we are talking about dysregulation of neuronal connections. The good news is that healing changes are possible thanks to the fact that the brain is malleable; it has the capacity to change and establish new connections, even in an adult. This quality is called *neuroplasticity*.

We have found that certain interventions that gently stimulate the brain through sound, light, electricity, or other modalities can affect neurochemicals and brainwave pattern. This stimulation can positively and safely improve neurological function. Collectively, I call these interventions *neuromodulation*.

What Is the World Like for a Child With Autism?

A child with autism experiences the world in a different way. To better understand some of the most important brain dysfunctions of autism, I invite you to attempt to experience with me the world as a child with autism might experience it.

First, let us look at language problems. Imagine you are traveling to a foreign country where people speak a language that you do not understand at all. You go to a crowded area, perhaps a mall or a marketplace.

How difficult would it be to decipher and understand what is being said with all the commotion around you?

This cacophony of strange sounds gives you an idea of how an individual with autism may experience language.

Now let us look at sensory stimulation. Imagine being next to a very loud siren or an alarm that goes off. You are unable to move yourself away from the situation; in fact, you are forced to move even closer to the source of the alarm.

That's going to irritate you, right?

This is what some kids with autism experience. Certain auditory stimuli that we can tune out may be extremely loud and annoying to them.

Finally, often we will see children with autism flap their arms or flap their hands; we call this *self-stimulatory behavior*.

You may look at this behavior from the outside and think: *That is bizarre.*

Put yourself in the mind of this child.

Why might you be making these movements?

If you have a motor dysregulation, you might be having difficulty finding your arm in space. Imagine how this might feel to you.

Can you see how moving your arms around several times may help you to establish where your limbs are in space?

Another possibility is that you might be experiencing an uncomfortable amount of excess activity in your brain and the repetitive movements work to quiet down that activity.

Hopefully these examples have given you an idea of what may be going on inside the head of a child with autism.

In addition, you may not be aware that more than 30 percent of children with autism also have seizures. These can range from silent or subclinical to severe seizures that may not respond to conventional anticonvulsant therapies.

These issues, in combination with behavioral problems, anxiety, and other areas of dysfunction, force us to look for innovative treatments that work safely. In our practice, we use various tools to address all the above, including special diets such as casein-free/gluten-free, specific carbohydrates, and ketogenic. We use pharmaceutical-grade dietary supplements or nutraceuticals, and a variety of neuromodulation interventions — transcranial direct current stimulation (tDCS), neurofeedback, photobiomodulation or laser treatment, and cranial electrical stimulation, or *Alpha*

Stim. We collaborate with gifted therapists who provide various rehabilitative therapies such as occupational therapy (OT) speech therapy, and Masgutova neurosensorimotor reflex integration (MNRI). We also use cannabidiol (CBD) hemp oil, which is a form of *medical marijuana.*

CBD oil is used to:

- Regulate abnormalities
- Reduce inflammation
- Enhance neuroimmune function
- Maintain homeostasis

Psychosocial and Spiritual Factors Play an Important Role in Autism

We have discussed some of the various clinical and biological processes and abnormalities that are found in children with autism and related disorders. However, there are other factors that are just as important and must be addressed. These are the psychological, social, and spiritual factors that are critical parts of the Restoration Model.

Imagine a young couple who are expecting their first child. They have high hopes. The child is born and appears healthy, but a couple years later, that child stops progressing, becomes delayed linguistically, loses the ability to make good eye contact with the parents, and later on — after a lot of turmoil and several visits to the doctor — receives the label of *autism*. This can lead to feelings of despair, dismay, confusion, and other unpleasant emotions.

The Restoration Model asserts that some factors that lay outside of the concrete biological realm also play a role in the health of a child with autism. Psychosocial factors and spiritual factors should also be addressed.

By spiritual, I'm not referring to religion. I'm talking about deeper issues regarding life:

- What is the meaning of life to you?

- Why has *your* child been afflicted with autism?

- What does it mean for your lives that this has happened?

- Does it matter clinically if you have hope?

- How does optimism in a parent, caregiver, or teacher factor into the progress of a child with autism?

- What effect does pessimism in caregivers have?

If you have a child with autism, don't discount these spiritual elements. They have a vital role to play in the biological and mental health of any child. For everyone involved, cultivating the right attitude is invaluable. Develop the fortitude that is needed to work persistently with a child. Going the extra mile can make all the difference.

When you are looking for treatment for your child with autism, be sure to partner with the right type of provider, physician, or therapist. Seeking out individuals who are committed, compassionate, and caring, as well as educated and skilled, will better enable your child to find healing.

Understanding Biopsychosociospiritual Interactions Is Key

Humans have been endowed with complex and powerful mental abilities and this makes any neurological disorder significant, and potentially difficult to treat.

We are also multifaceted beings:

- We are *biological* beings with some purely biological functions and needs.

- We are *social* beings with a need to communicate and emotionally connect with each other.

- We are *psychological* beings with unique minds, personalities, and thought patterns.

- We are intensely *spiritual* beings.

The complexity of any neurological disorder is, in part, due to our multifaceted nature. It follows that we should look at all four of these spheres—biological, social, psychological, and spiritual—as working in unison, although at any particular time we may selectively and artificially choose to focus on just one area.

Complex disorders that are resistant to even the best biological interventions available may simply require that we look at all the above areas to find where a solution may lie. We must first acknowledge that these different spheres of function are all disrupted by complex illnesses. Then, understanding the various interactions that exist between these realms can enhance our understanding of how to solve complex medical—or should we say *human*—problems.

Spiritually, we all have different qualities and outlooks. Some people may feel more fulfilled than others, or may have a more constructive outlook on life in the face of adversity. Some may seek spiritual virtues such as love and compassion that can affect mental as well as biological functions. A person's spiritual outlook can deeply affect their health and their recovery from illness.

Addressing the biological, the psychological, the social, and the spiritual as a unit can make a huge difference, since every part interacts with the other. This is the foundation of our Restoration Model.

The Restoration Model

The tenants of our model are:

- Biological disturbances can lead to disorders that are best understood in the biological or physical realm.

- Psychological disturbances can lead to disorders that are best understood in the psychological or mental realm.

- Mood disturbances can lead to disorders that are best understood in the emotional or affective realm.

- Spiritual disturbances can lead to disorders that are best understood in the spiritual or transcendental realm.

- Social disturbances can contribute to disorders that are best understood in the social or communal realm.

- The Restoration Model acknowledges the complexity and multifaceted nature of the human experience.

- In addition to disturbances that are best explained by the various realms and their respective constructs, important interactions exist between each realm. For example:

- A biological disturbance such as a brain tumor, a palpable abnormality, can result in seizures, which are a physical disorder.

- A brain tumor at the same time can cause personality changes that are intangible.

- The presence of a brain tumor and the physical and neuropsychological changes it causes can lead to secondary problems that involve the spiritual realm.

- Total healing is predicated on properly addressing all abnormalities in each of the human facets or spheres while also fine-tuning interactions between them.

CHAPTER TWO

Alzheimer's Disease
Treating a Brain-Mind-Behavior Nightmare

ALZHEIMER'S DISEASE: REFLECTIONS ON MEMORY, COGNITION, AND BRAIN HEALTH

Alzheimer's disease is a devastating condition that primarily affects the senior population. However, by studying this condition, we can cultivate a better understanding of memory and cognitive functions for people of all ages. We can learn more about what needs to be done to keep the brain healthy.

In the last chapter, we discussed autism, which is a childhood-onset condition that also affects the brain in many ways. Autism and Alzheimer's disease have a few other things in common. They're both sex-dependent, in that there are three to four times more cases of autism in males than there are in females, whereas Alzheimer's disease is more common in females than males. In addition, there is a gene called *activity-dependent neuroprotective protein* (ADNP) found in patients with both conditions; this may be a link of significance between these two important disorders.

Alzheimer's Disease Allows Us to Appreciate Memory

As a child neurologist, I have worked primarily with children, and especially with autism. But in the past few years, I have also been working with adults, including those with Alzheimer's disease. The level of suffering is tremendous for patients and their loved ones. You may not appreciate the importance of memory until you start experiencing the effects of memory loss. It can be completely devastating.

So it was for a patient back in the 1890s whose name was Auguste Deter. This individual, who was initially normal, started experiencing memory loss and began screaming for hours at night. She had sleep problems and was in an intermittent vegetative state.

But in a few moments of lucidity, the patient stated, "I have lost myself."

She was admitted to a mental institution, and the physician who evaluated her was Alois Alzheimer. Auguste, then, was the first patient diagnosed with Alzheimer's disease.

Alzheimer's is a complicated disease that is often hard to treat, just like autism. We know that it degrades memory, which is a complex function of the brain.

There are many different types of memories; they can be classified in different ways.

For example, memory may be classified as:

- Long-term
- Short-term
- Immediate
- Procedural
- Declarative

There is a specific process that allows new memories to be added to the brain. This process can be disrupted, as in the case of people with *anterograde amnesia*, who may forget information that is freshly presented. For example, they may read headline news that is groundbreaking, and then ten minutes later, they may have to read the same thing over because they have forgotten what they have just read.

Alzheimer's disease involves progressive loss of memory which is one of the most recognized symptoms of Alzheimer's disease. *Semantic memory*, where context-independent information is stored, such as names of colors and other basic facts, and *episodic memory*, which stores information specific to a particular context, such as time and place, are both forms of memory that can be consciously recalled or declared — hence the term *declarative memory*. Declarative or *explicit* memory — a form of long-term memory — starts to be affected early during the course of the Alzheimer's disease. Over time, *working memory* — a form of short-term memory involved with immediate conscious perceptual and linguistic processing — is also impaired.

Memory is valuable and any problems with memory will strongly impact quality of life. It can devastate not only the person experiencing memory loss, but loved ones who care for this individual.

Alzheimer's Represents a Group of Conditions That Are Associated With Dementia

You are probably somewhat familiar with Alzheimer's disease, and that is because it is present in up to 60 to 80 percent of the dementia cases that are diagnosed. Besides Alzheimer's, there are various other conditions that can present with dementia. These include vascular dementia, Huntington's disease, Parkinson's disease, frontotemporal dementia, dementia with Lewy bodies, and Down syndrome.

What is interesting from the above examples — which represent only a partial list — is that some of these conditions can start quite early. For example, young patients with Down syndrome may develop dementia, and Alzheimer's disease can affect middle-aged adults. Frontotemporal dementia may present as early as in the twenties, although most individuals with this condition have dementia in their forties, fifties, or sixties.

Some of these dementias present not only with memory loss, but also with changes in personality, interpersonal relationships, and conduct. They can affect every area of the victim's life.

Because it may take years for a person to become aware that they may have a medical problem, it may be quite some time before they look for treatment. A person in their forties diagnosed with a dementia-related illness may have exhibited marital problems and other interpersonal abnormalities for years without understanding that these were symptoms of their illness.

What is behind these changes in memory and cognitive function?

Brain Health: Principles for Improving Brain Function in Neurological Disorders

Many patients in my practice—children and adults—come to me looking for a different approach, in terms of helping brain function, memory, or various neurological or neurodegenerative disorders, including

Alzheimer's, Parkinson's disease, and autism. What I have found in my years of practice is that there are certain principles that can be beneficial in designing a strategy to help the brain improve over time.

First, it is important to properly diagnose the condition, along with all the underlying areas of dysfunction that may be present. To diagnose a condition accurately, we need different types of investigative tools.

Here are some methods that we commonly employ for diagnosis:

- Metabolic blood and urine tests
- Nutritional blood tests
- Hormone level assessments
- Tests for food allergies or sensitivities
- Toxicological urine tests
- Stool tests to evaluate gastrointestinal health and test for *leaky gut syndrome*
- Neuroimaging
- Electroencephalogram
- Genetic testing

The earlier we can assess a patient, the earlier we can intervene to treat an illness and keep it from progressing. In some cases, early genetic testing can allow us to implement preventative treatment. In the case of Alzheimer's disease, for example, early genetic testing can show if someone may be predisposed to

Alzheimer's disease. That individual may require early nutritional therapies focused on reducing or preventing inflammation, promoting levels of antioxidants in the cells, and avoiding or protecting against dangerous toxins. In these cases, we may be able to intervene early enough to prevent the disease from happening in the first place.

What about treatments?

Medications by themselves often may not get the job done and can cause significant side effects—almost as bad as the problem being treated in some cases, or sometimes even worse. When it comes to alternative interventions, there is an assortment of safe and effective tools that can be used.

These therapeutic tools include the use of specially selected foods for a patient. I call them *brain foods* or *food for thought*. This kind of *nutritional neurology* can be employed to address the toxic load in the body and brain, which is a problem commonly found in neurodegenerative disorders like Alzheimer's disease.

Nutritional therapy can help these patients in many ways:

- Some foods help to reduce inflammation, which is now recognized as a final common pathway in many chronic and neurodegenerative disorders.

- Some nutrients can boost mitochondrial function, which is often impaired in these conditions.

- Nutritional therapy can help fine-tune hormonal imbalances that may coexist with the neurological condition.

- Adjusting the diet is an essential part of treating any associated gastrointestinal issues.

- Nutritional neurology can help adjust immune or neuroimmune disturbances.

- Nutritional therapy can enhance neuromodulation methods, which will be discussed further in a later chapter.

Did we leave anything out?

Yes! Remember that psychosociospiritual factors are also important and cannot be ignored. They should be part of every comprehensive treatment plan. Two such factors to consider are stress and trauma.

Stress has been shown to affect neuronal function in an adverse way. Hormonal activity and the immune system are also negatively affected by stress. Patients with Alzheimer's disease and other brain disorders can benefit greatly from stress-relief strategies. Indeed, removing or reducing stress for a patient who is undergoing cognitive changes may be more effective than anti-dementia drugs. In addition, consider how stress affects the support system of each patient; family members and loved ones can also benefit from stress-relieving activities.

As a holistic medical provider, I do my best to identify any traumas that may have triggered or contributed to the onset of neurodegenerative symptoms. These traumas may be multiple, or they may be cumulative in their effects. They may be recent events or may have started decades earlier. They can be biological, but also psychological, social, or spiritual. Whatever their nature or origin, traumas that impact the patient's state of health should be identified and addressed as part of the healing process.

If you are struggling with memory problems, brain fog, or other cognitive impairment, or if you have a loved one with Alzheimer's disease or a related condition, take comfort. *It is not too late* to attain optimal brain health. Lives distorted by neuronal degeneration can be restored. As long as there is breath, there is life.

SEEKING THE CAUSE OF NEURODEGENERA-TIVE CONDITIONS

Alzheimer's disease is by far the most common cause of dementia. As such, the disease has had a serious impact on our population and on our healthcare system.

Suffering from Alzheimer's, as we have discussed, can be a heartbreaking struggle. It is also devastating for friends and family when someone who has been normal for decades suddenly starts to suffer from memory loss, along with changes in personality.

It is crucial for health professionals to try to understand why neurodegenerative conditions such as Alzheimer's disease and Parkinson's disease occur. Because we know that memory is affected by Alzheimer's disease, and because we know the parts of the brain where memory resides, we can focus on studying these areas of the brain in an effort to try to understand the factors and triggers that are damaging to them.

As we learn more about the process of memory storage and loss, with diligent study and research we can figure out how these processes are affected by conditions like Alzheimer's. Understanding how these diseases affect the brain, as well as all the other factors that are involved in brain health and recovery, will help us to create effective treatments.

Alzheimer's and Environmental Toxins

For many years now, people have wondered if there might be a connection between environmental triggers and the development of neurodegenerative conditions such as Alzheimer's disease. Researchers have found that heavy metal toxins such as aluminum play a big role in Alzheimer's disease. There may be various other environmental triggers as well.

We find that toxins like these affect not only patients with Alzheimer's disease, but also those with other neurodegenerative conditions, such as Parkinson's disease, and even conditions in the pediatric population, such as autism. It has been found that many children with autism have difficulty getting rid of heavy metal toxins, like aluminum and mercury.

Please see the following links regarding research publications from MIT and other institutions:

- people.csail.mit.edu/seneff/Entropy/entropy-14-02227.pdf

- ncbi.nlm.nih.gov/pubmed/23609067

Alzheimer's and the Accumulation of Reactive Oxygen Species

Medical researchers, for many years now, have noted that some reactive oxygen species — also called *free radicals* — can cause significant damage to various tissues in the body. There are various chemical reactions in the body that create free radicals as a by-product, and these must be neutralized. The way to neutralize these free radicals is by antioxidants.

In this discussion of neurological disorders, we are interested in the effects of free radicals on the brain. In the brain, interestingly, several important and necessary reactions, such as the production of neurotransmitters themselves, can lead to the production of free radicals, making it a necessity for the brain itself to have strategies to neutralize them.

Unfortunately, over time, due to a variety of factors, the body may have difficulty keeping up with the demands necessary to neutralize the free radicals with antioxidants. The use of antioxidants is recognized as being key to helping with brain function and for providing protection against the damaging action of free radicals that can lead to neurodegeneration.

Free radicals can be produced in excess when *mitochondria*, which are largely responsible for energy metabolism, function abnormally in our bodies' cells. Because mitochondria are implicated in a variety of neurodegenerative conditions, an active part of our strategy in my clinic is aimed at supporting mitochondrial health and promoting proper functioning.

Alzheimer's and Nutritional Neurology

We know that there are certain nutritional changes or abnormalities that can have a profound impact on various brain functions, including memory. It follows that proper nutrition and specific dietary interventions can play an important role in Alzheimer's disease and various other neurodegenerative conditions.

As far as nutritional neurology, we should consider that in some patients, there might be a deficiency in key nutrients that are needed for proper brain function.

Examples include:

- B vitamins
- Vitamin D
- Zinc
- Copper
- Magnesium
- Iron
- Fats

B vitamins are important for many functions, including the formation of neurotransmitters and the support of mitochondrial activity. Vitamin D, we now know, is more than a vitamin; it is also a hormone. Vitamin D receptors, in fact, are found throughout the body, including in the brain. Therefore, they play an important role in various neurological disorders, including Alzheimer's disease. Vitamin D is also important for immune health and diabetes.

Minerals such as zinc, copper, and magnesium are needed for cognitive function as well as for immune and neuronal regulation.

Iron is a vital for body functioning. If a patient has low iron in the blood, this can lead to restless leg syndrome and other sleep problems. This in turn can lead to chronic sleep deprivation. Sleep allows the body to rest and heal. Sleep deprivation, when chronic, is a powerful disruptor of health and recovery. Supplementing with iron can, in many cases, help with quality of sleep. When sleep is normalized, the immune system can be strengthened so that active healing, which often occurs during sleep, can be reactivated.

Just like iron plays a vital role in the body, there are other nutrients that support various health functions, including:

- B vitamins, such as B12, folate, and B6. These play an important role in energy production, cellular metabolism, and synthesis of neurotransmitters.

- Minerals and trace elements, such as magnesium and zinc. These are important for brain, mental, immune and gut health.

- Vitamin D. This vitamin is important for mood, brain and bone health, immune function, and various other functions, since virtually all cell types in the body have vitamin D receptors.

- Antioxidants, such as glutathione and alpha lipoic acid. These nutrients provide protection from oxidative stress, liver detoxification, and many other crucial functions.

But let's not forget about lipids—fats—that are also necessary for the health of the nervous system. We know that essential fatty acids play an important role in brain functions, including memory and cognition.

Fats have been criticized for being bad for the heart and arteries, but when it comes to the brain, fat is good! In fact, the brain is made up mostly of fat, and it is necessary for healthy functioning. Of course, nutritionally, it is good to manage our diets so that they primarily contain good, healthy unsaturated fat, like coconut oil, avocados, and fish, such as salmon and sardines.

The other aspect of nutritional neurology is the recognition that certain food items are harmful to the brain, causing sensitivities, allergies, or worse, severe brain toxicities. We know that gluten, for example, can cause significant inflammation of the brain and gut for those who are susceptible. Even healthy individuals who are asymptomatic may be experiencing transient leakiness of the gut caused by gluten.

Addressing nutrition and diet can play quite an important role in brain health and in conditions such as Alzheimer's disease. As a nutritional neurologist, I know that food matters. Nutrition often serves as the fundamental starting point in addressing brain restoration.

WE CAN SLOW AND EVEN REVERSE NEURODE-GENERATION WITH THE RIGHT APPROACH

Neurodegenerative conditions, especially severe ones, represent a group of conditions that, sadly, are often resistant to conventional medical interventions. Many people suffering with these neurodegenerative disorders have not found a good treatment solution that can slow down the progression of their disease, let alone stop or reverse the damage. Most conventional physicians treating these conditions end up simply trying to control symptoms by using a variety of medications.

What if I told you that there was a treatment modality, or set of principles, that could drastically impact brain function, even in disorders such as Alzheimer's?

Would you believe that was possible?

When I was a medical student, I also enrolled in a graduate program. This was a newly established interdisciplinary health and humanities program that I was invited to join at Michigan State University in 1990 as the first dual-degree medical student.

I had the opportunity, as part of a thesis project, to work with a large variety of nonallopathic — meaning nontraditional — providers and doctors, including chiropractors. I learned that they often took care of medical cases that had not been successfully addressed within the conventional or traditional allopathic model. They were there to provide hope to patients with chronic problems when the conventional system failed them. Often, they were successful in helping these patients.

As an integrative neurologist today, I feel the same way. Many of my patients come to me for help after having seen conventional doctors who have failed to solve their problems. They are looking to me for different strategies for treatment. They are looking to me for hope.

Always Address Gut Health First

As a conventionally trained neurologist, I was taught that there was a set of questions that a neurologist should always ask while trying to solve neurological problems:

"Where is the abnormality?"

"How long has this problem been there?"

And so on.

Now, as an integrative neurologist and functional medicine specialist, I have learned that the first question to ask is, "What is going on in the gut?"

I always remember the phrase: *As goes the gut, so goes the brain.* It is true in many situations.

In our gut, we have up to 100 trillion bacteria that form what are called *microbiota*. The genes the cells harbor are called the *microbiome*, although the terms microbiome and microbiota are often used interchangeably. Gut microbes are important in that they can influence your mood, memory, and other neurologic and mental functions.

How can this be?

Gut microbes produce neurotransmitters and hormones identical to those produced by humans and can therefore send signals to the brain via the vagus nerve. These signals can influence various brain-related functions, as mentioned above, and also influence sleep and stress. See the following link: ncbi.nlm.nih.gov/pmc/articles/PMC4259177/.

As we have already discussed, the functioning of the gut affects the other systems of the body. We should always make sure that the gastrointestinal system is working well when dealing with brain disorders. Two common conditions that may be of concern are *gut dysbiosis*, in which there is an imbalance of good and bad bacteria, and *leaky gut syndrome*, in which the internal lining of the intestines becomes porous and allows toxins to go into the blood system.

How are gut issues related to neurological issues?

Here are some examples:

- Gastrointestinal problems often exist concurrently with neurological disorders.

- The functional problems that cause leaky gut syndrome sometimes may also cause the so-called *leaky brain syndrome*, which can account for brain fog and memory issues.

- Inflammation of the gut can be associated with localized immune dysregulation, since 60 to 80 percent of immune cells are found lining the gut. Immune dysregulation can significantly impact neurological function, as you will read in a later chapter.

- Having healthy gut bacteria, or *flora*, can result in the release of important neurotransmitters and anti-inflammatory mediators from the beneficial gut bugs.

- A sick gut can spell trouble for the brain, since an overabundance of bad gut bugs can lead to these organisms releasing *neurotoxins* or toxic substances that are harmful to the brain.

Addressing Environmental Toxins and Toxins Within the Body

One of the many lessons I have learned after spending years working with children with autism is that if someone has a problem with toxins, these toxins can adversely alter function in the brain and other parts of the body, such as the intestines, liver, and other organs. For children with autism, as you have read, removing these toxins can lead to significant improvement in neurological and overall function.

What do we know about toxins?

- We know that toxins can take many forms.

- Some body toxins involve microorganisms. For example, yeast and bacteria can release toxins that can go to the brain, bypassing the blood-brain barrier, causing trouble.

- Toxins can take the form of heavy metals; we have already talked about aluminum and how that plays a role in Alzheimer's disease and autism.

- Toxins can come in the form of pesticides and herbicides. For example, in the agricultural product Roundup, the chemical *glyphosate* is thought to be associated with many disruptive symptoms including leaky gut syndrome.

- When it is working properly, the body has natural detoxification mechanisms.

- There are genetic mutations and variants that can prevent proper detoxification from taking place.

- When they are not eliminated properly from the body, toxins can inhibit different brain functions.

- The presence of some toxins in the body and brain can lead to behavioral, mood, motor, sensory, cognitive, movement, and emotional disturbances.

Proper Utilization of Nutrition and Neuromodulation

In terms of using nutritional neurology to help the brain, it boils down to an understanding of proper nutrition, which entails intake of the right foods — and possibly dietary supplements — that will influence the neurochemistry of the brain. We want to improve the functioning of the brain by fostering the restoration of proper activities, prompting a return to the normal regulation of neurotransmitters and other neurochemicals.

We also must consider what we call neuromodulation. Before I talk to you about neuromodulation, I'm going to talk to you about *neuroplasticity*. Neuroplasticity refers to a quality that the brain possesses — the quality of being able to adjust in response to changing conditions.

When I was in my first year of medical school, I took a neuroscience course. In it, I learned that the brains of children are neuroplastic, but most of that plasticity was lost by adulthood. I was so disturbed by that information that, right then and there, I decided that I would not go into adult neurology, but child neurology. I reasoned that because the brains of children were still malleable, I might be able to have a greater impact by working with children than I would with adults.

Much later I learned that even the adult brain is neuroplastic. Moreover, I also learned — contrary to what I was taught in medical school — that the brains of children and adults have the capability to grow new brain cells through a process called *neurogenesis*.

We know today that neurogenesis can be enhanced by antioxidants found in some foods — especially those containing flavonoids such as blueberries — and omega-3 fatty acids. Neurogenesis can also be influenced by other factors, such as aerobic exercise and the brain activity that comes from learning new things. On the other hand, neurogenesis can be slowed down by stress, inflammation, alcohol, and a high intake of saturated fat.

The bottom line is that we can rewire the brain by incorporating appropriate lifestyle changes. We can also use a process called *neuromodulation* to improve brain function. Therapeutic neuromodulation is the alteration of nerve activity through the delivery of electrical, sound, light, or other forms of stimulation or chemical agents to target sites of the body.

Examples of neuromodulation devices that we have found useful include:

- Cranial electrical stimulation or Alpha Stim
- Photobiomodulation, which uses low-level lasers
- The Brainwave app, a simple pocket tool that can be downloaded to your smartphone
- Neurofeedback
- Transcranial magnetic stimulation
- Transcranial electric neuromodulation

We are currently planning on using a next-generation device that combines dense array EEG, a form of high-level electrodiagnostic testing, with Geodesic Transcranial Electric Neuromodulation (GTEN).

In our practice, we have found that incorporating neuromodulation interventions can greatly enhance brain function in young children with autism, as well as in seniors with Alzheimer's disease. Neuromodulation, coupled with good nutrition, can produce drastic improvements in patients.

I hope this chapter has helped you understand that if you or a loved one — adult or child — are suffering from Alzheimer's disease, Parkinson's disease, Huntington's disease, or another neurological problem, there are treatments that can work, even if you've been told otherwise. Positive changes can be made to enhance your quality of life. In addition, if you are healthy right now, steps can be taken to make sure you remain that way throughout life.

Using the Restoration Model, we look for treatments that address the specific needs of each individual patient. We assess patients comprehensively according to the proper principles and design targeted interventions, including neuromodulation and nutritional therapy.

CHAPTER THREE

PANDAS
A Brain-Immune-Psychiatric Disorder in Children

PANDAS: DESCRIBING THE BRAIN-IMMUNE CONNECTION

PANDAS, or *Pediatric Autoimmune Neuropsychiatric Disorders Associated with Streptococcal infections,* is an ideal condition to help us describe the brain-immune connection.

We have previously discussed the concept of the three brains. First, there is the intracranial brain — the gelatinous glob inside our skulls. The second brain is the intra-abdominal brain, composed of the set of nerves and neurons that control and regulate our digestive system; and the third brain, the floating brain, is also known as the immune system. This mobile brain is versatile, but complex. It is protective of our bodies, but, in worst-case scenarios, can antagonize one's own cells.

In this chapter, we are going to focus on the immune system. We will look at PANDAS and some other conditions that highlight how important the immune system is.

PANDAS Is a Neuropsychiatric Immune Nightmare

Imagine a healthy eight-year-old boy named Johnny. He is well-adjusted, well-behaved, healthy, and intelligent. Then, overnight, this child starts to behave differently. He gets irritable, he becomes very anxious, he obsesses over a lot of things, and his cognitive skills are regressing.

The first impulse of Johnny's parents is to take him to his primary care doctor. The doctor examines him and finds nothing wrong. It is suggested that he may need to see a psychiatrist. This seems like good advice to the parents at this point because Johnny, a previously docile and calm child, has turned into a little monster. He has started to attack his parents, he is no longer in control of his emotions, and he has severe rages that would cause any parent to cry. He obsesses over strange things and seems very anxious. To his parents, Johnny is no longer the same child they had a few days before.

The psychiatrist immediately treats Johnny with a cocktail of powerful antipsychotic medications, but the child does not get better; in fact, Johnny gets worse. Now he starts having motor tics; that is, involuntary movements, so the child is sent to a different specialist, this time a child neurologist.

The neurologist looks at Johnny and suggests that the child may have Tourette's syndrome, a tic disorder that starts in childhood and is often accompanied by other symptoms, including neurobehavioral and mood problems.

The neurologist prescribes an anti-tic medication and another medication to help with focus and attention, since these have also become problem areas. That is not the end of it. Johnny is sent to a urologist because he now urinates excessively for no apparent reason. Johnny continues to deteriorate.

What is going on?

This is a realistic description of a child who has developed the condition called PANDAS. This is a brain-immune condition in which the patient's own antibodies attack a part of the brain called the *basal ganglia*. This results in a broad range of neuropsychiatric changes that significantly impair a child's quality of life. There is no better example of a devastating condition that affects immune, neurologic, and psychiatric function at the same time.

PANDAS Highlights the Consequences of a Dysfunctional Immune System

When it comes to our health, there are many things that we tend to take for granted. One of these is our immune system. As we've stated, the immune system is quite complex. It employs an elite surveillance system that keeps us protected from harm. It also commands a daunting defense system, much more powerful than any army.

As you may imagine, regulation of this system is of paramount importance. PANDAS is a condition that allows us to have a glimpse of what can happen when the immune system becomes dysregulated; you can get any number of abnormalities that can cause horrific pain, both physical and emotional.

When the immune system is dysfunctional, problems can arise in any part of the body. As a neurologist, of course, I am primarily concerned about neurological functions.

If the immune system malfunctions, what effect can this have on the nervous system?

As a result of immune abnormalities, a whole host of neurological problems can arise, including:

- Abnormal movements
- Mood changes

- Anxiety
- Cognitive changes
- Fine motor problems
- A decline in handwriting skills

Conditions like PANDAS illustrate how important the immune system is. We should do everything we can to strengthen and protect it, and do what we can to ensure that it remains well regulated.

PANDAS Demonstrates How an Immune Dysfunction Can Alter Mental Function

Several years ago in my practice, I started getting referrals from some psychiatrists who were sending me young patients with a variety of psychotic and mental problems. You might think this to be an odd type of referral because as neurologists, we tend to focus on neurological abnormalities instead of psychiatric ones.

So why were these psychiatrists referring these children to me?

They had become aware that PANDAS could be an explanation for some cases of abrupt mental illness in children. Children with this disorder often have sudden changes of mood, severe anxiety, obsessive-compulsive behavior, or panic attacks. Commonly prescribed antidepressants, antipsychotic medications, and even cognitive therapies often don't work for these patients. Because PANDAS is a neuroimmune disorder, if this diagnosis is suspected, a psychiatrist may suggest a referral to a neurologist.

In some cases, conventional treatments may be effective. Usually, however, if you have a child who has an autoimmune problem such as PANDAS, the best approach is to focus on re-regulating the immune system. In these cases, when you help the immune system function normally, the child's brain function, mood, and overall mental wellness are more likely to improve, quickly and safely.

THE IMMUNOLOGICAL COMPONENTS OF BRAIN DISORDERS

What I have learned over the past several years is that, when confronted with a complex neurological case, I must take a step back and not just focus on the nervous system, but also assess what is going on with the immune system.

In fact, truth be told, in evaluating a new patient, I am likely to spend about one-third of my time talking about the brain and the nervous system, another third of the time talking about the digestive system, and the last third of the time talking about the immune system.

The reason is that there are a variety of immune disturbances that will secondarily affect the brain and cause what may present as a primary neurological problem, but in reality are immune-initiated disturbances that secondarily affect the nervous system. These patients will require immune-modulating interventions for successful treatment.

The Nervous System and the Immune System Are Intimately Linked

Most scientists and clinicians would agree that the brain and the nervous system are the most important of the organ systems in the body.

I am not just saying this because I am a neurologist and am biased in favor of my field. We all realize that without a brain, the human organism cannot function at all. We also recognize that the brain is a very complex and delicate organ.

It follows that we need an immune system that is robust, ready to protect and defend every aspect of the nervous system.

Scientists have discovered that certain cells located in the brain actually play a significant role in immunity themselves. In the past, it was thought that the brain had two main types of cells: the *neurons*, which are active and involved in thinking and other brain processes, and a second type called *glial cells*, which were thought to be mainly physically supportive cells.

Now we know that these glial cells are also active participants in neurological functions, including neuroimmune activities. Glial cells can destroy pathogens directly with minimal damage to healthy brain cells and can switch on various processes, including inflammation. This illustrates, among other things, the close relationship that exists between the immune system and the nervous system, and the fact that if one system suffers, then the other one may not function optimally.

Assessing the health of the immune system in patients with neurological issues is a key part of the Restoration Model. By considering that a neurological or neurospsychiatric disorder may have an underlying immunological deficit, even if not apparent at first blush, we can maximize the chances of treating these disorders successfully.

Immune Dysfunctions Can Lead to Structural Brain Damage as in Multiple Sclerosis

Multiple sclerosis is one of the most devastating neuroimmune disorders. It is caused by an immune disturbance that results in physical and structural changes in the brain and in other body parts.

Common findings that are suggestive of multiple sclerosis involve what doctors call *neurological symptoms separated in time and space*. An adult who was previously healthy and active may suddenly begin to experience intermittent symptoms. Perhaps that individual may lose vision in one eye, and then may recover, but then may have weakness or tightness of one limb. Then, at a later date, balance may be disturbed.

Often, if you scan the brain and spinal cord of individuals with multiple sclerosis, you will find abnormalities in different locations. These are what doctors call *lesions*. The lesions reflect damage to the insulating myelin lining of the nerve cells. This damage is due to a disturbance in the immune system that has resulted in an attack on the patient's nerve tissue.

Some other immune-mediated disorders can affect brain function and lead to structural abnormalities. Celiac disease, for example, is a condition in which gluten may not be tolerated and may cause an abnormal immune response. In the case of celiac disease, just as in the case of multiple sclerosis, there may be structural changes in the brain that can show up in magnetic resonance imaging (MRI) of the brain. Celiac disease can also cause problems with walking or gait — a condition called *gluten ataxia* — and a whole host of other problems.

Hard-to-Control Seizures Respond to Specific Neuro-immune Treatments

Seizures affect about 0.5 percent of the U.S. population. When seizures occur out of the blue, as they often do, this can lead to a lot of distress; it is a very scary phenomenon. Neurologists are aware that a certain percentage of individuals with recurrent seizures, or what we call epilepsy, will not respond to conventional pharmacological treatment; that is, medications may not stop the seizures. What is interesting to note is that in a subset of these individuals, using immune-modulating treatments, such a steroids or intravenous immunoglobulin, can stop the seizures.

Further research shows that in some cases, the immune system can attack the brain, launch an assault, and cause symptoms like seizures. To stop the seizures in these cases, the patient needs some immune-modulating treatment. This, again, is an illustration of the intimate connection between the immune system and the nervous system.

Learning about the brain-immune connection, as well as the brain-gut connection discussed earlier, helps us understand more fully that the body works as a unit — all parts are interconnected in sickness and in health.

Looking at the body this way when assessing a patient may be critical to successful treatment and, in some cases, it may be life-saving.

RE-REGULATION OF THE IMMUNE SYSTEM CAN RESULT IN BRAIN RESTORATION

When dealing with a neuroimmune problem, we should proceed with an understanding that the immune system, when working properly, is a great asset, but when dysfunctional it becomes instead a powerful, destructive force. Our primary strategy, in these cases, should be to *re-educate* the immune system; in other words, to re-regulate or reprogram the immune system so that healing can occur.

Neuroimmune Interventions Can Have a Dramatic Effect on Neuropsychiatric Disturbances

It is most gratifying to see, in conditions such as PANDAS, when a child who has spent several months — and in some cases, *years* — suffering from a variety of neuropsychiatric symptoms finally gets relief. Coming up with the right treatment protocol can make such a difference in the lives of these children, and sometimes very quickly.

In the case of PANDAS, treatment with antibiotics often can lead to quick resolution of symptoms. In more severe cases, use of intravenous immunoglobulin can be highly effective. It has been shown that, without a doubt, re-regulating the immune system can help to resolve neurological symptoms, from anxiety and mood changes to movement disorders such as tics. There are also cases resembling PANDAS that are not caused by a bacterium like strep, but are caused by a virus instead. We call this *Pediatric Acute Onset Neuropsychiatric Syndrome* (PANS). These may also respond to antibiotics.

PANS, Antibiotics, and Neuroimmune Regulation

PANDAS is a subtype of the broader PANS. Unlike PANDAS, which is specifically associated with the bacterium Group A Strep (GAS), PANS does not require an association with GAS. It is a clinical diagnosis and can be associated with various other infectious agents. These include atypical bacteria such as mycoplasma pneumonia, Lyme disease—a tick-borne bacterial illness—and viruses, such as influenza and varicella.

Even in PANS where the inciting organism may be a virus, when treated with antibiotics, a PANS patient can respond quickly with full remission, in some cases in as little as one to two days on antibiotics, though it often may take longer, up to two to six weeks. For further elaboration on the criteria and guidelines for PANS and PANDAS, please refer to the PANDAS

Physicians Network (PPN), a group that maintains clinical guidelines for PANS and PANDAS (pandasppn. org/what-are-pans-pandas/).

The question is how can a viral-induced PANS patient respond to an antibiotic when these are commonly thought to be useful only for bacterial infections?

The answer is that studies show that antibiotics themselves have a direct central nervous system function. They can improve neuropsychiatric symptoms, and they also have immunomodulatory effects. There are several research articles on this topic.

For a great example that is well referenced, I refer you to the 2012 article by Dr. Obregon and colleagues entitled, "Psychotropic effects of antimicrobials and immune modulation by psychotropics: implications for neuroimmune disorders" (ncbi.nlm.nih.gov/pmc/articles/PMC3494283/).

Introduction to Cannabidiol (CBD) Oil and Immune Regulation

As we have mentioned above, the immune system is powerful, but when it becomes dysfunctional, it can cause all types of difficulties and lead to a variety of brain-related disorders. Scientists have discovered a critical system in the body, called the *endocannabinoid* system, and have found that this is one of the most pervasive systems in the body. By pervasive, I mean that all body systems are regulated by this all-important communication network. This includes the nervous, musculoskeletal, respiratory, cardiovascular, digestive, reproductive, tegumentary (skin), endocrine (hormonal), and immune systems. This is why the uses of CBD oil are so broad. It brings everything into internal balance, or what we call homeostasis.

There are receptors peppered throughout the body that interact with the endocannabinoid system. When this system in your body is working well, you can remain healthy. When this system is disturbed, it can lead to a variety of illnesses.

Cannabidiol (CBD) oil acts on receptors found in the brain, immune system, and other parts of the body and is known to have broad functions ranging from pain control to an anti-nausea and anti-tumor effect. As far as the brain is concerned, CBD oil works well for seizures, even those that are medically refractory to medications and other modalities such as the ketogenic diet and vagal nerve stimulation. Tzadok and colleagues have reported phenomenal results with CBD oil in a multicenter trial in Israel (involving five pediatric epilepsy clinics) in a paper published in 2016, "CBD-enriched medical cannabis for intractable pediatric epilepsy: The current Israeli experience" (ncbi.nlm.nih.gov/pubmed/26800377).

CBD oil is also found to be safe and effective for psychiatric problems, including psychosis and schizophrenia. For further information, I recommend a 2012 paper by Zuardi and colleagues, entitled, "A critical review of the antipsychotic effects of Cannabidiol: 30 years of a translational investigation" (*Curr Pharm Des.* 2012; 18(32):5131–40). In addition to neurological and psychiatric conditions, CBD oil has been found to be useful for controlling nausea and vomiting, anxiety, chronic pain, and sleep perhaps in part because CBD oil has anti-inflammatory and antioxidant functions (ncbi.nlm.nih.gov/pubmed/21238581).

As I started using CBD oil in my practice, I discovered that it can be a useful adjunctive tool for helping people feel better and recover, even in difficult cases. The endocannabinoid system also helps to manage inflammation, and assists in immune regulation. So here again we find evidence that, if we can reeducate the immune system, healing can occur.

Controlling Inflammation and the Use of Antioxidants: Improving Immune Function

Many chronic illnesses have a final common pathway that involves inflammation. When there is inflammation in the body, it can cause disruption and dysfunction of tissues throughout the body. One of our strategies, therefore, in helping to treat chronic illnesses and other problems, including neuroautoimmune difficulties, is to control or eliminate inflammation altogether.

We are finding that many chronic and complex disorders may secondarily involve a system in the body called the *mitochondrial system*. The mitochondria are small organelles inside of the cells that are the powerhouse of the cells; that is, they produce energy. By supporting the mitochondria, we support the immune system by allowing healing to occur faster. Antioxidants and proper nutrition, as we have discussed already, are key to mitochondrial health.

A general strategy for health and healing should include gaining control of inflammation, nourishing the body with a strategic selection of nutrients and antioxidants, and applying other interventions that will have the overall effect of improving immune function.

If you are a patient, and you are suffering from a chronic condition, perhaps you have already been seen by multiple physicians and specialists, yet you are not getting better. Please consider the fact that your immune system may be involved, but also consider that your gastrointestinal system may be perturbed, and so may your nervous system.

In fact, it is a big mistake to consider all these different organ systems as working separately. One key point is the understanding that all these systems are closely intertwined and intimately linked.

To find healing, you should always think of these three main systems — the nervous system, the immune system, and the gastrointestinal system — as working together. Also take into account associated organs and systems, like the liver, the lymphatics, and the hormonal apparatus. By supporting the health of each one of these, we can bring the body back into balance and harmony, and healing may ensue.

CHAPTER FOUR

Schizophrenia
The Ultimate
Psychiatric Disorder

UNDERSTANDING THE MIND AND MIND-BODY INTERACTIONS

I have a younger brother, now thirty-six years old, who became mentally ill at the age of eighteen after a nervous breakdown. I have seen up close what it's like to deal with mental illness and the mental torture that it can entail. In fact, this experience has allowed me to understand how a person can be fine when the mind is working appropriately, but when that is no longer the case, it is almost like a living hell. We sometimes take the mind, like the immune system, for granted until it stops working properly.

In this chapter, we will explore the mind-body connection. We will look at mental illness and psychosomatic interactions. Above all, we will explain why people who suffer from mental illness can be assured that there is hope; that with the right understanding and the right treatment approach, mental illness can improve, and even go away. I hope that you, the reader, will pay close attention to our discussions in this very important chapter.

The Mind Is a Reflection of Brain Health and Vice Versa

The brain is a fragile, gelatinous organ inside the skull that is the control center of the entire body. An important function of the brain is the generation and management of thoughts, language, and other intangible constructs that we call collectively *the mind.* Many view the brain as the organ of the mind. For sure, there are a lot of experiences that fall in the realm of mental phenomena, and it is a complex relationship, but it is certain that we need a well-functioning brain to have a well-functioning mind. The two are linked.

When you consider the physical organs in the body, you can probably easily understand that if you have a broken bone or you are bleeding, your body does what it can to heal the injury. The same applies to the mind. If the mind is traumatized by an event, the mind tries to repair what is dysfunctional.

We know that the same processes that are used to explain healing in a physical sense can also be applied to healing of the mind. Both can be bruised and traumatized, and both, with the right approach, can be healed. There are even medical interventions that can assist, such as Eye Movement Desensitization and Reprocessing (EMDR), which is a type of psychotherapy that can assist in the recovery of a traumatized brain, utilizing something akin to Rapid Eye Movement (REM).

Although Mental Phenomena Are Complex, They Follow Specific Laws

In order to understand the laws that apply to mental health, it is important to understand that we have both a conscious mind and a subconscious mind.

The subconscious mind, it is said, is responsible for the overwhelming majority of mental activity, perhaps over 90 percent. This does not mean that the conscious mind is not important. It is the conscious mind that allows us to focus and to attend to activities at hand. In doing so, it may sometimes restrict our ability to perceive and conceive certain ideas, while there is no such limitation in the subconscious mind.

This is important to understand, because—just as in the case of the brain or other tissues—what we feed the mind can eventually affect our mental health. It is important to guard our mind, both the conscious and the subconscious.

Everything we've ever said, done, or experienced is stored in the subconscious mind. This information can be tapped into, hopefully in a positive manner, to help us heal a suffering conscious mind.

We do have some specific principles that apply to mental health. If these are understood and used properly, they can promote wellness and bring happiness.

Mental Health Is Intimately Related to Brain Health

One of the individuals who fascinated me as I started to learn about the brain and mental function when I was in college was a doctor by the name of Dr. Wilder Penfield. He was a famous neurosurgeon who was born in the United States and lived in Canada. In the 1950s, he started to do brain surgeries for epilepsy and other conditions. He would always take the time, before he started to operate and while he did the surgeries, to stimulate certain parts of the brain.

He would use local anesthesia so that the patients were actually awake during the surgery. Although the bone, the skull, and the *meninges* — the tissue covering and protecting the brain — all have pain fibers, the brain itself has no pain fibers, and does not feel pain. So, before Penfield started cutting the brain, he stimulated different parts of the brain without causing pain to the patient. It turns out that things that had been seen, felt, and experienced a long time ago could be brought back to the surface with the help of electrical stimulation. It's interesting to note that when he, for example, poked at the temporal lobe, people were able to recall different experiences.

He found that the experiences ranged from simple — for example, hearing a voice — to very complex, and even mystical, such as out-of-body experiences. So, we know that the mind and the brain are very much linked. Even in the case of near-death experiences, the brain may appear completely dysfunctional, but people have vivid otherworldly experiences.

Trauma sometimes causes changes to the mind. There was a man named Phineas Gage who, in 1848, had a severe brain injury. He was using a tamping iron that, unfortunately, went through his cheek and through his skull, and completely altered his personality. He went from a quiet, calm individual to one who became very aggressive. His was, in fact, the first reported case that showed a link between brain trauma and personality change.

The mind and the brain are also linked to the immune system. A field called *psychoneuroimmunology* is dedicated to the study of the way feelings and perceptions can affect our immune function, which in turn can affect the way our nervous system works.

As a medical student, I participated in some research in the field of psychoneuroimmunology and found it fascinating to explore the relationship between the brain, the immune system, and the mind.

Clearly, the mind and the brain are intimately linked. Because of this close relationship, we know that if we can make the brain healthy, the result can be improved mental health.

MENTAL ILLNESS AND PSYCHOSOMATIC CONDITIONS

Back in the late 1990s, I was at the University of Cincinnati on a training fellowship in neurology. I took care of a young lady who was in her early thirties. She came in the emergency department having convulsions and seizures. These were so severe that she received high doses of intravenous anti-seizure medications. The seizures did not stop, so she required multiple doses of these medications.

I was on call, so I was contacted and decided to admit her to the neurology service. We gave her further medications. At that point, things were getting desperate; it had become a life-or-death situation. The seizures weren't stopping and she had been convulsing nonstop for hours; this is a serious condition called *refractory status epilepticus*.

The team and I decided to take her to the intensive care unit so we could induce a *pentobarb coma*, which sometimes is used to stop recalcitrant seizures. Then I saw that some tears were flowing out of her eyes. I instinctively asked if she was okay, which is not normally done when someone is having seizures, since they're not aware of their surroundings.

I was stunned when she answered me. Because she was sedated, she only mumbled, but it was clear that she was conscious and could hear me. It then dawned on me that she was not having true epileptic seizures, but what we call *psychogenic seizures* — stress-based seizures — for which we were about to induce a coma, which would have been a mistake. This experience demonstrates how powerful mind-body interactions can be in causing severe disorders that appear to be neurological in clinical presentation but are stress-related in their origin.

Understanding Mental Disorders and Psychosomatic Conditions

Conditions such as schizophrenia, depresson, and bipolar disorder, although complex, are often better understood than psychosomatic conditions.

Consider the example that I gave above, of the lady who presented as an epileptic patient but turned out to have an emotional disturbance. These cases can be confusing. In fact, let me take the time to briefly explain certain terms. *Psychosomatic*, or mind-body problems, belong to a class of conditions in which mental or emotional conflict has been converted into bodily symptoms or issues that appear neurological.

In contrast with psychosomatic conditions, there are various additional terms that are applied to disorders that appear physical or neurological but for which no underlying physical pathology can be found.

These terms include:

- *Conversion disorder*, a term that was coined by Sigmund Freud, in which an underlying stress-based problem *converts* unintentionally — the patient is not faking — to a neurological symptom. A more modern term is *functional neurological symptom disorder*.

- *Somatic symptom disorder*, previously called *somatoform disorder*, is a new, broader term encompassing disorders where *somatization* occurs — that is, mental phenomena that are expressed as physical or somatic symptoms due to mental distress.

The main difference between psychosomatic disorders and somatic symptom disorder is that the former results in actual physical abnormalities that can be measured objectively, while the latter is subjective.

Sometimes we use the term *psychogenic*; that is, something that is generated in the mind. *Malingering*, on the other hand, would be akin to faking an illness.

Mental disorders or psychiatric conditions are disorders that reside predominately in the mind—disorders affecting thoughts—unlike conditions that start in the mind's *psyche* and secondarily also cause bodily or somatic symptoms, earning the label *psychosomatic disorders*.

Understanding the differences between all these is important, but in every case, the mind is involved in some way. Sorting out the mind-body question and fully defining psychosomatic abnormalities are difficult tasks. However, we know that if we attend to the mind, as well as the brain, and we address these issues for patients in a comprehensive manner, we can help both brain and mind to function optimally.

Psychosomatic Problems Lie in the Borderland Between Brain and Mental Function

In the world of medicine, we tend to classify conditions and have them addressed by different specialists. For example, psychiatrists will work with mental disorders, although they originate in the brain. Neurologists will deal with neurological problems, although there may be a mental component.

However, there are conditions that lie in what I call *the borderland between the mind and the brain*. These conditions involve symptoms and processes that do not fit neatly within the neurological realm or the psychiatric realm. In these cases, we must try to understand the conscious mind and the subconscious mind, as well as the functioning of the brain pertaining to the mind. It is in this *borderland* that many psychosomatic illnesses arise.

Psychosomatic problems may be related to stress, or to traumatizing events that are meaningful to a particular individual. We know that most visits to primary care doctors are, in some way, stress-related. If we can manage our stress properly, this can have a dramatic effect in reducing psychosomatic illnesses that often are poorly understood by the medical profession.

Differentiating Between Psychosomatic Abnormalities and Psychiatric Disturbances

As I mentioned earlier, I have a younger brother with a psychiatric condition. He has been diagnosed with schizophrenia. However, when I have analyzed his condition over the years, I have found it hard sometimes to differentiate between behavioral symptoms that are due to a true psychiatric condition and those that might be psychosomatic, or even under his volitional control.

In reality, psychogenic, psychosomatic, and mental illnesses may overlap tremendously. It is important, therefore, in tackling these problems, to make sure that we keep our focus on restoring and maintaining a healthy brain and a healthy mind.

In terms of mental function, we can think of it as good mental hygiene when we do activities — like meditating and using pure thoughts — that can feed our minds in a positive manner. Similarly, we can foster brain health by providing nutritional elements, as we will discuss below, that will help the brain to function optimally. While it can be difficult to distinguish psychosomatic abnormalities from purely psychiatric or mental problems, treating these conditions holistically can result in improvement for all patients.

REVERSING MENTAL ILLNESS IS POSSIBLE USING SPECIFIC PRINCIPLES OF THE RESTORATION MODEL

In the United States and around the world, there are many individuals who are suffering with mental illnesses. In a sense, mental disorders may be more difficult to deal with than purely physical problems, because when you have a mental illness, you are dealing with a condition that is *invisible*. When you go for a medical evaluation, there may not be any specific physical abnormality that shows up on a brain scan or on other tests.

Individuals with mental illnesses may feel alienated and may be stigmatized. Much suffering is associated with these disorders. Studying how best to approach the minds and mental function of patients can lead us to an effective plan for treatment and healing. Only then can quality of life improve, not just for the patient, but for family members as well.

Understanding the Causes of Mental Illness Is Crucial

We have found that mental illnesses can be understood using the principles of the Restoration Model, which is predicated on a comprehensive bio-psycho-social-spiritual approach.

In some cases of mental illness, there may have been traumatizing events that have disrupted mental function, leading to the illness, but there may also be genetic factors.

For example, Dr. Kenneth Plum has discovered a specific mutation in the dopamine receptor (DRD2) that is associated with a number of problems, such as addiction, alcoholism, obsessive-compulsive disorder (OCD), and anxiety.

There are other genes like the so-called *warrior* gene — the monoamine oxidase A (MAOA) gene — that has been associated with aggression and other behavioral changes. We also know that infections can cause sudden changes in behavior; we discussed one example, PANDAS, in an earlier chapter. These are just a few examples of conditions that, if properly identified and treated, can lead to healing and wellness from a mental health perspective.

Stress is a significant factor in mental illness. We see many instances in which a mental disorder may have had its onset following a stressful and traumatizing event. We also know that stress can exacerbate a mental disturbance that already exists.

Part of any treatment strategy, therefore, must be to recognize the importance of stress for patients, and to help them learn to cope with it in an efficient and effective manner.

Like Neurological Disorders, Mental Illnesses Respond to Dietary Interventions

We know that every cell in the body, including brain cells, requires proper nourishment to function optimally. When it comes to mental illness, it turns out that if we can feed the brain and feed the body, we are, in essence, also feeding the mind. For this reason, I call proper nourishment *food for thought.*

There are certain nutrients—vitamins, minerals, and antioxidants—that can help improve not only brain function, but also mental function, and in some cases even reverse mental illness altogether.

We find, for example, that vitamin B12 deficiencies can affect not only brain cell function in the form of a neurological disorder, but mental function as well.

More than ten years ago, I took care of a young boy who had started experiencing hallucinations. He appeared to have what looked like a religious experience; he was prophesying the end of the world and preaching on street corners. At the same time, it was noticed that his eyes started turning yellow, and he became very pale. One day he abruptly fainted in the middle of the street where he was prophesying. When taken to the hospital and examined, it was found that he had a dangerously low vitamin B12 level. After getting injections of B12, these problems quickly went away, and he was restored to health.

There are numerous other examples of nutritional connections to mental health. It is important to factor in nutrition when dealing with mental disorders.

If you are a patient under the care of a psychiatrist, and you have been placed on psychotropic medications, but you feel that you are not getting better, then consider the role of nutrition in your mental health. You may want to find a good functional medicine doctor who can guide you in the use of nutrients — essential fatty acids, omega-3 fatty acids, and antioxidants — that can bring healing for your brain and your mind.

Neuromodulation: A Missing Link in Many Cases of Hard-to-Treat Mental Illness

As I have mentioned earlier, individuals who have mental illnesses suffer tremendously, as well as family members and caregivers, especially in the case of hard-to-treat conditions. For that reason, I want to offer you information on special tools that are available and can be implemented in addition to medications that you may be taking for a psychiatric problem.

We've already talked about the role of nutrition and dietary interventions for mental illness. In addition to these, neuromodulation may be of great benefit for patients with conditions that are difficult to manage.

Neuromodulation treatments are based on the principle of *neuroplasticity*; that is, the brain is malleable and capable of change. Even in an adult, brain cells can make new connections. If the brain can be properly stimulated, these new connections can also help improve mood disorders and other aspects of psychiatric function.

Neuromodulation devices can be useful as an auxiliary tool to help with mental illness, and even stress. Below are some techniques and tools that are commonly used, including ones that we employ in our office.

- Psychiatrists and neurologists have been using a device called TMS, which stands for Transcranial Magnetic Stimulation. This has been shown to be beneficial in the treatment of refractory or resistant depression.

- In our office, we use a technique called TDCS, or Transcranial Direct Current Stimulation. We can place electrodes in specific areas on the scalp to provide directed stimulation that can help with problems like anxiety, depression, mood, and various other difficulties.

- There's a device called Alpha Stim that is cost-effective and portable that can also help with stress and mood problems.

- There are even neuromodulation devices that are inexpensive, such as the Brainwave app that can be downloaded on an iPhone or Android.

We know that maintaining a healthy brain is necessary for the mind to operate properly, and vice versa. The use of a broad, holistic, wellness-based approach that addresses the bio-psycho-social-spiritual elements of every individual can help restore and maintain a healthy mind and brain. This is the aim of the Restoration Model.

I hope that the information in this chapter has helped you see that there are an assortment of tools that can be used if you or a loved one is suffering from a mental disorder or psychiatric condition. You do not have to continue suffering.

Work with a provider who can incorporate the different tools that are available, and who will address your particular needs so that healing can occur. Don't give up!

CHAPTER FIVE

Fibromyalgia
Understanding Functional Illness

FUNCTIONAL ILLNESSES ARE OFTEN POORLY UNDERSTOOD AND MISDIAGNOSED

Functional illnesses are conditions that plague many individuals. First, let us define what a functional illness is. By definition, a functional illness is a condition that cannot be diagnosed based on a well-defined biological mechanism of action. Likewise, testing may not reveal an abnormality that accounts for the illness at hand based on conventional evaluations. The cause may be unknown, although stress-related factors often play a role. Functional illnesses may have an acute onset, but the symptoms tend to be chronic.

As you can imagine, having a disorder that is not detectable by examination or by laboratory testing can pose problems, and it does. Many such patients are not taken seriously, and therefore they suffer without getting the help that they need. As a functional medicine neurologist, I have seen many of these patients over the years, both children and adults, and have found that they can be helped.

Is It All in Your Head?

People who are suffer with functional illnesses are often told, "It's in your head."

In a sense, all mental or neurological disorders are *in the head*, aren't they?

This includes many of the functional disorders. That is not to say, however, that they are not real and cannot cause significant impairment to the quality of life.

A good example of a functional illness that is fairly common is *fibromyalgia*.

Many individuals are plagued by this condition, which can cause:

- Pain
- Discomfort
- Chronic fatigue
- Chronic abdominal pain
- Irritable bowel syndrome
- Noncardiac chest pains

Many years ago, I trained with a neurology professor who was very by-the-book and traditional. He often referred to fibromyalgia as *get-a-life syndrome*. He thought that fibromyalgia was a condition that was completely in the person's head and nothing more. He thought it was a waste of his time to take care of such individuals. I suspect he adopted that attitude merely because he did not have the right tools or framework to have a better understanding of the disease and how to address it.

Fibromyalgia is an interesting condition to discuss, and it is a good one to use as a representation of functional disorders in general, since it is common.

How do we treat this kind of disorder?

Using the principles of the Restoration Model, symptoms can be improved by using the bio-psycho-social-spiritual approach that we have discussed.

Specifically, we can target the symptoms from several perspectives:

- Fibromyalgia is associated with many different symptoms, as described above, and these symptoms are associated with different body systems.

- Biological interventions, such as removing gluten from the diet, can be helpful.

- Neuromodulation intervention, such as biofeedback, neurofeedback, transcranial direct current stimulation, or Alpha Stim, can be effective.

- Interventions that address mental function, such as relaxation, meditation, and stress management, can have a huge impact.

- Having a strong support system that includes family members, relatives, the community, and society in general can have a strong psychosocial impact.

- Finally, spiritual matters are also important; we must ensure that a patient's ultimate sense of belief, value, meaning of life, and purpose are taken into account.

Functional Illnesses Are Often Not Identifiable by Abnormal Test Results

Medical doctors and specialists have become overly reliant on tests, and at the same time, often ignore the environmental context and belief system of a patient, and other factors that may be important to health.

Tests should be an adjunct in the medical diagnostic process; they are only one part of a complete assessment of the patient. Note that a normal result on a test does not rule out the presence of a disorder. It also does not preclude the existence of serious disease.

When it comes to lab results, there is a so-called reference range within which a *normal* blood or urine test result is considered acceptable by conventional doctors. Unfortunately, this range may be at times quite broad and may not reflect what is *optimal* for a patient. As such, a blood test may come back *normal* but, in reality, that lab value may be far from *optimal* and from what is required for health. This means that a patient may be given a lab result and may be told that everything is fine — with a vitamin D level or ferritin, for example — when, in reality, the level is below what is needed for healing to occur. That area — suboptimal vitamin D level — may not be addressed for that patient and can limit optimal care that is needed. This problem, where *normal* is confused with *optimal*, is a common one and sadly can delay a patient's return to full health.

Given the above, it is important for physicians to be good listeners and understand what patients are trying to say, even if what is said does not fit neatly into a conventional medical box — and even if the test results are negative. Health providers are there to take care of their patients.

Health Providers Often Offer Little Hope to Patients Suffering From Functional Illnesses

In many cases, patients with functional illnesses, such as fibromyalgia, adrenal fatigue, or chronic fatigue syndrome, are frustrated by visits to their conventional doctor. They often leave the office having little hope that they will ever feel better. Sometimes, these patients may not feel like they have been understood. They may even feel that the provider didn't believe that they were having true symptoms.

This is complicated by the fact that even family members of a patient with a functional illness may think that they are making up their symptoms to some extent. To them, their loved one simply isn't behaving in a way that is consistent with a true medical problem; symptoms might be vague or variable, or simply invisible to the observer.

When tests come back with normal results, they seem to confirm the fact that the patient doesn't have a real illness. This is why many functional illnesses can take many years to diagnose. It is very important, therefore, for such individuals to find the right type of medical provider in order to get appropriate help. The good news is that such help exists.

FUNCTIONAL ILLNESSES ARE AS REAL AS MORE ESTABLISHED MEDICAL CONDITIONS

Just because a condition does not present in a neatly packaged and well-defined manner — according to pre-existing, conventional medical guidelines — this in no way means that the problem is not a real or important medical condition.

Some diseases that are functional with obscure etiologies may become better understood in the future and may be identifiable clearly by tests at that point. In any case, a health provider should be there to help you if you are a patient who has come to them for assistance.

Using the Restoration Model, we can approach the symptoms of these functional illnesses in a comprehensive manner. We begin with a discussion of gut function.

There Is a Link Between Gut Function and Functional Illness

We have previously discussed the importance of gastrointestinal (GI) health, and the fact that the gut is at the crossroads of all major systems, including the nervous system, the immune system, and the digestive system. Therefore, there are many contributors to functional illnesses that involve gastrointestinal abnormalities.

You may recall that in the GI tract, there are more than a hundred million nerve cells and 60 to 80 percent of our immune cells lie in the digestive system. In addition, lining the inner digestive tract, we have what are called *tight junctions* that protect against pathogenic bacteria and toxins. If these toxins were to cross into the bloodstream, due to lack of proper protection, this could lead to devastating consequences.

It is often confusing and frustrating when a patient who suffers due to a medical problem, such as fibromyalgia with diffuse pain, brain fog, and significant fatigue, goes to several medical specialists and, after a lot of testing, is told, "we cannot find anything wrong."

Similarly, a child who has hard-to-control seizures — despite taking appropriately prescribed anticonvulsant medications — and whose brain scans and other labs do not provide an answer is left without hope. The same holds for the individual who is becoming forgetful and irritable without medical explanation.

What do these have in common?

They may all potentially be explained by and successfully be addressed based on an understanding of how the gut works and how gut-related abnormalities can result in illness. Importantly, addressing gut dysfunction can lead to restoration of health in many patients with enigmatic disorders that fall in the realm of functional illness.

Let us look at gut problems and their relationship to functional illnesses in more detail.

All of us have varying amounts of good, healthy, and beneficial bacteria in our gut that regulate digestion and other gut functions. The more abundant these bacteria and the more diverse they are, the better. They also contribute in an important way to our overall health. It is this realization of the connection between beneficial gut bacteria and overall health that has led to the increased popularity of taking oral probiotics in the past several years.

Unfortunately, there are other types of bacteria that also reside in our gut that are less beneficial and may in many cases cause harm to the body. These gut bugs are called *pathogenic* bacteria. An imbalance between beneficial and pathogenic bacteria in our colon, or gut dysbiosis. This gut dysbiosis can result in a variety of symptoms involving not only the gut, but also the brain and immune systems.

Beneficial bacteria can release a host of products that can influence the brain— neurochemicals similar to those released by neurons in the brain, control inflammation and oxidative stress (e.g., butyrate), and provide many other useful functions, while pathogenic bacteria may release toxins that adversely affect brain and immune function.

Intestinal Permeability or leaky gut syndrome is another condition in which the tight junctions that we mentioned above become compromised, causing a leakiness of the digestive tract, allowing gut bugs, antigens, toxins, and other foreign materials to enter the bloodstream. Dr. Alessio Fasano, gastroenterologist, researcher, and chair and division chief of gastroenterology at Mass General Hospital in Boston, is well known for his work on leaky gut syndrome and gluten. Leaky gut syndrome from gluten can also cause *leaky brain syndrome* thanks to dysregulation of a protein called *zonulin* that regulates the opening of tight junctions in the gut and extra-intestinal cells affecting the blood-brain barrier.

One of my favorite examples is *gluten ataxia*. This is a condition where ingestion of gluten in some predisposed individuals can result in an autoimmune reaction to gluten, in which antibodies attack the cerebellum causing *ataxia* or balance problems and difficulties walking.

If you are a patient who is suffering and about to give up because you are not finding answers, you may very well have a functional illness. To change your situation, you should start by asking if you have leaky gut syndrome or gut dysbiosis.

Is your brain fog a result of leaky brain syndrome?

Then ask yourself if your doctor is addressing these gut-related problems.

If not, where can you find a medical provider who can address these problems so you can reclaim your health again?

Fortunately, a growing number of clinicians are being trained in functional medicine, where these issues are studied in detail for the benefit of patients who are looking for safe solutions to their medical problems.

Toxicological Problems and Functional Illnesses

When it comes to functional illnesses, there is a growing recognition that toxins can play a major role.

Some common types are listed below and will be discussed further in the paragraphs that follow:

- Environmental toxins
- Yeast toxins
- Bacterial toxins
- Mold toxins
- Toxins produced by the body itself

A variety of different toxins exist, and they can harm different tissues in the body. Earlier we mentioned an herbicide product called Roundup that contains an ingredient called glyphosate, which can cause an assortment of problems in many people. Other environmental toxins, such as organophosphates (PCBs for instance), beno(a)pryrene, and many others, have received a lot of attention regarding health. When discussing the various causes of functional illness, it is important to always address the possible presence of a toxic exposure and one's innate ability to clear the body of these toxins, to detoxify.

Yeast can release toxins that can cause symptoms, as can bacterial pathogens. Mold is another big issue, especially black mold and other types that produce neurotoxins. These can have devastating effects.

Finally, under conditions of *endogenous toxicity*, toxins may be produced from within the body due to a variety of abnormal metabolic defects. One such condition is called *adrenoleukodystrophy*. The movie *Lorenzo's Oil* depicted a boy with this condition. It is caused by the body's own production of very long chain fatty acids that can accumulate into toxic quantities.

Another form of endogenous toxicity can be due to metabolic byproducts of gluten, which is found in wheat, and casein, which is found in dairy products. Many children with autism, for instance, have an inability to properly break down and process gluten and casein. Their dysfunctional metabolism creates opioid-like products like *gluteomorphin* and *casomorphin*, which can have toxic effects on the brain. These effects may account for some of the behavioral problems that we see in these children, such as hyperactivity, irritability, and self-stimulatory behaviors.

Functional Illnesses Are Treatable and Respond to Specific Interventions

If you are an individual with a functional illness such as fibromyalgia, chronic fatigue syndrome, irritable bowel syndrome, chronic pain, or many of the other conditions that fill this category, I want to let you know that there is hope. If your condition is approached in the proper manner — one that is holistic and integrative — then your symptoms should improve, often significantly.

To treat functional illnesses successfully:

- The patient, loved ones, and health providers must first understand that these conditions are real, and that a systematic treatment approach can result in dramatic improvements.

- As physicians — especially functional medicine physicians — we try to be good listeners. We try to be empathetic and to listen in a nonjudgmental manner. If your doctor is not behaving in that manner, it may be time for a second opinion.

- Next, assess gut issues, since these can lead to a lot of secondary problems. I have listed and discussed some of the gastrointestinal problems that can lead to other difficulties.

- If you have a functional illness, you must clean up your diet, and you can do this by eating wholesome, organic, live, whole foods. This must come first, before considering even the addition of dietary supplements.

- Supplements should be used properly — as *supplements* to a good, healthy diet.

- Treatment should be employed to remove toxins safely and gently from the body.

- The hormonal or endocrine system should be assessed, and if there are imbalances such as thyroid or adrenal dysfunctions, these should be addressed.

- Make sure that sleep is adequate; good sleep hygiene and getting enough rest are indispensible. This can allow your body to heal and the immune system to become robust.

- Check that the mitochondrial system, which is the powerhouse of the cells, is working properly.

- Finally, address stress, mental health, and spiritual concerns.

TESTING CAN REVEAL RELEVANT DYSFUNC-TIONS PERTAINING TO FUNCTIONAL ILLNESS

As I have discussed above, many functional illnesses may not show up in common laboratory tests, which makes matters difficult, especially for conventional physicians who rely on such tests. Fortunately, there *are* tests that are available, although not always well known, that can shed some light as to the underlying cause and contributing factors to various functional illnesses. We will, in the next few paragraphs, address these.

Genetic Panels Have Been Developed to Identify Genetic Causes of Functional Illnesses

In the past several years, the field of genetics has improved significantly. I remember when I was trained in the field of neurology, and even before that, in my training as a medical student, I was taught that I should do genetic testing for kids who were labeled FLK. FLK stands for *Funny-Looking Kids*. This is what we were actually taught. If someone looked a little bit strange or abnormal, that was enough of a justification to order a genetic test.

Today, I know that when dealing with functional illnesses, it is useful to do genetic testing, because we might find specific gene abnormalities or gene variants that can explain the predisposition for various symptoms that are found. For instance, one may have an abnormal genetic variant that can cause the person not to detoxify properly, and therefore they may accumulate toxins more readily than someone who does not have that variant.

In my practice, we use specific genetic panels to help in the diagnosis of functional illnesses. Because many of my patients may come to my practice already on different medications, I also do specific testing called *pharmacogenetic* testing to see if the patient is able to properly metabolize the drugs they are on or about to be prescribed, or if they have a gene variant that increases the likelihood that they may have side effects to different medications based on genetic makeup.

There are also genetic panels that are useful for functional illnesses in that they focus on a panel of genes that regulate the detoxification system. These pathways involve biochemical pathways in the liver that may be defective, leading to various disorders, ones that lead to immune dysfunction, for example. This type of information can help the medical provider focus on the removal of toxins in a very personalized manner.

Particular Neurometabolic and Nutritional Disturbances Are Associated with Certain Functional Illnesses

Several integrative physicians who do research have found that there are certain vitamins and minerals that, if low, can result in various functional illnesses, including ones that affect brain function.

Some of the most critical are listed below and a discussion follows:

- B vitamins
- Vitamin D
- Copper
- Zinc

It is well known that if one has a low B-vitamin level, that individual may have lack of energy and other symptoms, but in reality, various functional illnesses are directly linked to vitamin B levels that are low, whether it is B12, B6, or riboflavin. The explanation for this, at least in the case of functional illnesses that have neurological presentations, is that B vitamins are co-factors for neurotransmitters, so if these levels are low, your neurotransmitters may also malfunction.

B vitamins also play a role in the mitochondrial system, the powerhouse of the cells. If your B vitamin levels are low, this may mean that the mitochondrial system may not work as robustly.

Vitamin D also can cause problems when low and is linked to various functional disturbances, including:

- Cardiovascular problems, such as high blood pressure

- Gastrointestinal disorders, such as inflammatory bowel disease and Crohn's disease

- Immune disturbances (many immune cells have vitamin D receptors), such as respiratory tract infections in children and autoimmune disorders like rheumatoid arthritis

- Endocrine problems, such as thyroid dysfunction

- Systemic, such as fatigue and aches and pain associated with fibromyalgia

- Respiratory problems, such as asthma

- Brain problems, such as multiple sclerosis and cognitive problems

- Neuropsychiatric problems, such as mood problems like depression and seasonal affective disorder

Apart from the above functional disturbances, vitamin D is well known to be linked to kidney disease such as Fanconi syndrome, with loss of phosphate and other nutrients in the urine, skin problems, such as psoriasis, and of course bone diseases such as rickets and osteomalacia.

Vitamin D is important because most cells in the body have a vitamin D receptors, including immune cells, B and T lymphocyte — hence vitamin D's role in autoimmune disorders. Even brain cells — in the hippocampus and other parts of the brain — have these receptors, explaining the relationship of vitamin D with memory and other cognitive functions.

If you would like to learn more about vitamin D, I refer you to a book by Dr. Michael Holick called *The Vitamin D Solution*. Dr. Holick is one of the foremost authorities and leaders in the field of vitamin D research.

Finally, copper and zinc are important. Zinc plays a big role in sensory functions and processing of various enzymes in the body. In addition, high copper levels combined with low zinc — what we call a *high copper-to-zinc ratio* — can lead to a variety of functional illnesses, including mental illness.

Making nutritional and metabolic assessments of patients with functional illnesses is an important part of the healing process. If imbalances are identified and treated properly, this can significantly improve symptoms and accelerate the restoration of health.

Detoxification Impairments Play a Major Role in Functional Illness

We have already alluded to the fact that there are a variety of toxins that can affect bodily function. Now, I want to explain a couple mechanisms that can highlight how toxins can disturb bodily functions.

One of the main common pathways for chronic illnesses in the body deals with inflammation. Many toxins that accumulate in different parts of the body can eventually cause inflammation, and the underlying tissue may cease to function properly.

In the case of the brain, toxins that traverse the blood-brain barrier into the brain can cause, in time, *neuroinflammation*.

Because of this fact, it is important to highlight the need for protocols for detoxifying the body. In the case of heavy metals, treatments use the process of *chelation*, whereby heavy metals are removed safely from the body. This can lead to significantly improved health.

Note that when someone is trying to get rid of yeast or other microbes, one is also engaging in a form of detoxification.

I must point out that whenever detoxification protocols are used, in some cases, a *healing crisis* may occur. When this kind of detoxification reaction occurs, the individual may get worse before they get better. This is because the toxins are being mobilized in the body tissues before they are released from the body. In the case of yeast and other microbes, we use the term *Herxheimer reaction* to describe these symptoms.

Using dietary therapies and supplements in the right sequence and detoxifying the body in an orderly manner can minimize detoxification reactions.

It is then necessary to identify toxins the best one can, and then try to get rid of them as part of the healing process. This is a major part of treating functional illnesses.

The existence of functional illnesses should encourage doctors, in general, to think outside of the box to help a segment of the patient population that is in need and is suffering chronically. A broader, more expansive approach to healthcare is needed in treating functional disorders.

There can be sharp differences between conventional medical doctors and those who are more holistic and practice functional medicine. If you have a functional illness, you need to determine what will work best for you.

In Chile, a Westernized conventional healthcare system exists, but many indigenous people—the Mapuche, for instance — prefer a more original, local, and holistic model.

While they recognize that strengths exist in the Western conventional model, they value an integrative approach that incorporates one's belief system. Great importance is placed on the proper balance and equilibrium between the natural and spiritual world. Both healer and patient are linked together in the care of the patient and, therefore, are on the same page, which is conducive to healing.

The development of the functional medicine movement among integrative or wellness-based doctors and other medical providers will certainly provide hope to countless functional medicine patients who, at the same time, do not feel understood and are not given the right tools for restoration of health.

Conclusion

We have discussed a variety of disorders, from autism to Alzheimer's disease. I chose these conditions because they represent a wide range of disorders that affect many individuals of all ages. Whatever chronic illness you may have, I want you to remember that complex illnesses require a comprehensive and integrative approach.

The body itself is made up of different organs and organ systems that must operate together as a whole unit. As such, treatment strategies must involve taking care of the entire body. The Restoration Model approach is a bio-psycho-social-spiritual one that at once encompasses body, mind, and spirit. Psychosocial and spiritual factors should not be ignored. They contribute a great deal to health and wellness.

If you are suffering, the good news is that healing is possible. We already have a self-healing body, a *doctor within*. It only needs the right ingredients, fuel, and tools to carry out advanced restorative functions.

You need not worry. In fact, worry, anxiety, and stress themselves can be destructive. Your thoughts and emotions can affect your brain function, which in turn can affect your immune system. Negativity can, ultimately, weaken your immune system.

If you are sick, you can get well, but there are a few things that you must do. In fact, if you want to feel better starting within the next few weeks, I would like to challenge you to do the following:

1. You must change your diet. Eat wholesome, fresh, unprocessed foods that are organic. Consider removing gluten from your diet.

2. Make sure that your bowel function is normal. Consider taking a probiotic agent. You should keep in mind that you can also build up your gut flora through food sources or by drinking certain beverages. These include:

   - Kombucha
   - Kimchi
   - Coconut
   - Kefir
   - Tempeh
   - Miso
   - Sauerkraut

   These fermented foods have multiple benefits in that they also contain vitamins, minerals, other nutrients, and *prebiotics* — food source for bacteria in our gut.

3. You must manage your stress. Take time out for yourself.

4. Try to be moderate in all things and avoid excess.

5. Get plenty of sleep. You should get enough sleep so that you wake up easily in the morning and feel fully rested and in a good mood. If you wake up and are tired in the morning, it means that you did not get enough rest, or the quality of your sleep was inadequate. Melatonin, a natural sleeping hormone, may help if you have trouble sleeping. If you continue to suffer, it may be time to see a sleep specialist. Sleep is important.

6. Engage in physical, but also mental, exercise on a daily basis. By mental exercise, I mean activities that challenge the mind, such as learning a new language or learning to play a musical instrument.

7. Always have an attitude of gratitude. Avoid holding grudges. Be optimistic. Always try to be positive.

Above all, the message I would like to leave you with is one of hope; hope that healing is possible, even if several specialists have told you that your condition is not treatable.

If you have a problem that doesn't seem to have a solution, it may simply be that you have not been following the right approach. You may not be improving because you are operating within a system that is not conducive to healing. Look for a system that addresses all your needs as a whole person and you may find the answers.

Don't ever lose hope.

Next Steps

Total brain—and body—restoration is possible. Don't wait. Start your journey to recovery today. To learn more about our unique and innovative approach, come and join us in one of the free group workshops held every other month at our center.

The Brain Restoration Clinic is located in the Greater Charlotte Region in North Carolina, just over the border into South Carolina.

Address: 1040 Edgewater Corporate Parkway, Indian Land, South Carolina.

Do not hesitate to call our office at 704-541-9117 to arrange a one-on-one consultation.

Visit our clinic website at brainrestorationclinic.com.

Like us on Facebook at *Brain Restoration Clinic* to find more information on brain restoration, nutritional neurology, and the ongoing activities at the Brain Restoration Clinic.

The Brain Restoration Clinic is a division of Integra Wellness Center (IWC). You can visit the IWC website at integrawellnesscenter.com.

Brain Restoration Ministries is a 501(c)3 nonprofit organization supporting unique wellness-based research. Learn more at brainrestorationministries. com.

Let us assist you and be part of your journey to Total Brain Restoration!

About the Author

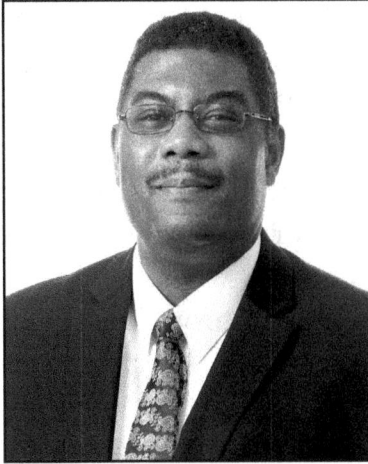

Dr. Corbier is a board-certified neurologist with special qualifications in child neurology. He works with pediatric and adult neurological patients. Over the past sixteen years, his focus has been on working with individuals with autism and related disorders using a special model he has developed, called the *Restoration Model*.

Dr. Corbier's Restoration Model is one of hope that brings comprehensive solutions to medical conditions that may appear enigmatic and untreatable. That is why he considers himself a *holistic* brain specialist, using an integrative biopsychosociospiritual- and wellness-based approach to help his patients with various complex neurological disorders.

Dr. Corbier earned his medical degree in 1995 from the College of Human Medicine at Michigan State University. He completed electives in neurology at Johns Hopkins Medical Center in Baltimore, Maryland, the Mayo Clinic in Rochester, Minnesota, and the University of Michigan. He also had the opportunity to study abroad for one summer in England at the University of London, where he focused on medical ethics and medical history. After completion of the graduate program, Dr. Corbier wrote a paper entitled, "A Biopsychosociospiritual Understanding of Mind-Body Interactions," that later became the basis in part for his current Restoration Model.

He completed an internship and pediatric residency at Michigan State University and went on to do his adult neurology training at the University of Cincinnati in Ohio, followed by a child neurology fellowship at the Children's Hospital Medical Center of Cincinnati, where he was the director of the neurology clerkship for medical students.

Dr. Corbier has been recognized for his work with autism and has been invited to speak at national conferences on this topic. He has been awarded the Patient Choice Award: Favorite Physicians in North Carolina for five consecutive years and the Compassionate Doctor Award for four consecutive years. He has shared his work on TV, radio, and through various lectures and workshops, and has authored several books and articles.

He is currently the medical director of the Brain Restoration Clinic, which is devoted to brain recovery using innovative, multimodal, and multidisciplinary approaches. The clinic is a division of the Integra Wellness Center (IWC), of which Dr. Corbier is also a co-founder. The IWC is a large center with multiple medical providers, specialists, and therapists.

Dr. Corbier serves on several boards, including Autism Speaks and the North Carolina Integrative Medical Society. He is also founder and chair of Brain Restoration Ministries, a nonprofit organization that provides free clinical care to indigent patients and supports medical research endeavors.

Dr. Corbier provides comprehensive, competent, customized, and compassionate care for his pediatric and adult patients and families. He also devotes one day of the week to wellness-based, clinical research.